Natural Therapies for Menopause

Practical, positive advice on diet, exercise, herbal remedies, osteoporosis, hormones, emotional problems, and much more!

Nancy Beckham

Keats Publishing

Chicago New York San Francisco Lisbon London Madrid Mexico City
Milan New Delhi San Juan Seoul Singapore Sydney Toronto

Library of Congress Cataloging-in-Publication Data

Beckham, Nancy.
    Natural therapies for menopause / Nancy Beckham.
      p. cm.
    Includes bibliographical references and index.
    ISBN 0-658-01221-5 (alk. paper)
    1. Menopause. 2. Menopause—Alternative treatment. 3. Naturopathy.
  I. Title.

RG186 .B425 2001
618.1'7506—dc21

2001029858

Keats Publishing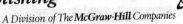

A Division of The McGraw·Hill Companies

1 2 3 4 5 6 7 8 9 0 DOC/DOC 0 9 8 7 6 5 4 3 2 1

ISBN 0-658-01221-5

This book was set in Centaur by Reider Publishing Services.
Printed and bound by R. R. Donnelley—Crawfordsville.

Cover design by Hebron Design
Photo courtesy of Eyewire

AUG 1 3 2002

McGraw-Hill books are available at special quantity discounts to use as premiums and sales promotions, or for use in corporate training programs. For more information, please write to the Director of Special Sales, Professional Publishing, McGraw-Hill, Two Penn Plaza, New York, NY 10121-2298. Or contact your local bookstore.

The purpose of this book is to educate. It is sold with the understanding that the publisher and author shall have neither liability nor responsibility for any injury caused or alleged to be caused directly or indirectly by the information contained in this book. Although every effort has been made to ensure its accuracy, the book's contents should not be construed as medical advice. Each person's health needs are unique. To obtain recommendations appropriate to your particular situation, please consult a qualified health care provider.

This book is printed on acid-free paper.

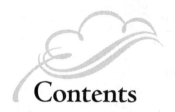

Contents

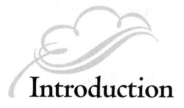

Introduction

$\mathcal{M}$enopause often coincides with the beginning of a new era in a woman's life. It is a transition period that may pass smoothly, inconveniently, or with difficulty, although menopause itself is not the main concern of middle-age women. In a survey of their health concerns, women ranked menopause symptoms at thirty-six of a list of sixty. Not surprisingly, stress, overweight, financial issues, and family problems topped the list.

Unlike the medical establishment, I do not consider menopause a disease, yet menopause is treated as a disease when hormone replacement therapy (HRT) is prescribed. All pharmaceutical drugs have benefits and risks, and in cases of serious disease, it is commonly accepted that the benefits outweigh the risks. Relatively healthy women, however, do not need to be exposed to the risks of HRT. In fact, the majority of women with reasonably healthy lifestyles will adapt to the lower level of reproductive hormones that their bodies supply during the nonchildbearing years. Some physicians are even debating the wisdom of prescribing hormones and are criticizing the standards and reporting methods of drug trials.

My recommendations are not as simple as swallowing a tablet. There are many foods, herbs, and supplements that will help you through the transition to a healthy postmenopause. Don't be disappointed if you have menopause symptoms or osteoporosis despite a healthy diet and lifestyle; many factors, including genes, can affect health. Sometimes the body simply needs additional support. I treated my own bones with natural remedies, and in one year I went from moderate levels of osteoporosis to normal. I recommend a high level of physical activity, more than a few strolls each week. In keeping with a naturopathic approach, I also suggest strategies for coping with stress and improving your inner self.

This book has five main purposes.

1. To explain why menopause is not a disease
2. To outline the reasons why healthy women should *not* take hormone replacement therapy
3. To give natural remedies for treating menopause symptoms and osteoporosis
4. To recommend what you should do to prevent osteoporosis and bone fractures
5. To suggest how you can live in harmony and health through and after menopause

The most important thing to understand is that there is much you can do to improve the length and quality of your life. The American Academy of Anti-Aging Medicine estimates that about 30 percent of the characteristics of aging are genetically determined; the other 70 percent is linked to lifestyle factors. Although economical disadvantage and poor education are reportedly the major risk factors for virtually all health problems, national wealth is not necessarily related to a longer, healthier life. In the United States, for example, the current life expectancy is 79.6 for women and 73.8 for men, which places Americans about sixteenth in the world. When the World Health Organization measured quality of life at age 70 in addition to length of life, the United States placed twenty-fourth in the world.

Although our bodies generally become less efficient as we age, it *is* possible to increase physical and emotional health. I see this increase in my clinic and yoga classes all the time. For most people, it's easier to make changes gradually. In time, you'll find you really didn't enjoy unhealthy food and harmful habits (well, most of them anyway).

It's never too late to improve your well-being and circumstances. Think of menopause as a stimulus for you to make beneficial changes.

CHAPTER ONE

The Menopause Experience

WHAT IS MENOPAUSE?

The word *menopause* means that your periods stop due to changes in hormones. In this book I use the word *menopause* to include the medical terms *climacteric* and *perimenopause* (the years immediately preceding and following the last menstrual period). Perimenopause includes the phase when periods may become erratic with possible heavy bleeding as well as flushing or other symptoms. Some women appear to have hormonal surges during this time and experience symptoms of excess estrogen or hormonal imbalances, which may be a sort of primordial reproductive urge innate in all living things. Postmenopause refers to the later years.

The Menstrual Cycle

From about ages twelve to fifty, women go through relatively regular menstrual cycles that are only interrupted by pregnancy, surgery, or illness. Estrogen and progesterone, which are secreted by the ovaries, are the main hormones involved, but their quantities and activities are controlled or modified by a number of other hormones. The levels of all these hormones are finely tuned from minute to minute and at different times of the menstrual cycle.

On day I of the menstrual cycle, the pituitary gland is stimulated by the hypothalamus in the brain to release follicle-stimulating hormone (FSH). This hormone is carried by the bloodstream to the ovaries where it stimulates follicles (egg sacs) to grow and secrete estrogen. The estrogen thickens the lining of the uterus in preparation for an egg that may be fertilized by male sperm. Once the estrogen levels reach a certain level, the pituitary gland is triggered by the hypothalamus to release luteinizing hormone (LH), which reduces the estrogen level and restricts the number of eggs that develop each month, generally to one. When this egg (the ovum) is mature, ovulation occurs; that is, it is released from the ovary and travels along the fallopian tube into the uterus.

The sac in the ovary that contained the egg develops into the corpus luteum (meaning "yellow body") and produces progesterone, which functions to thicken the lining of the uterus further and also to moderate the follicle's own continuing release of estrogen. This continues from about day 14 until a certain blood level of progesterone is reached, at which time the hypothalamus sends a hormonal messenger to the pituitary to stop secreting LH. The corpus luteum then shrinks and stops producing estrogen and progesterone. (If the egg is fertilized, however, the corpus luteum does not shrink and continues to produce relatively high quantities of progesterone to sustain pregnancy.)

If the egg in the uterus has not been fertilized, menstruation occurs once the levels of estrogen and progesterone have dropped to a certain level, and bleeding occurs around day 28 as the built-up lining of the uterus is shed. Then the cycle starts again.

Menstruating women have around fourteen days of high estrogen levels in their bodies and fourteen days of relatively high progesterone levels.

This hormonal interplay goes on for about thirty-five years, and its regularity varies. You know from your own observation that hormonal changes can result in various symptoms throughout your life cycle: acne at puberty, premenstrual irritability, period pain, and morning sickness during early pregnancy. The same principles apply at menopause except that the hormones undergo a major change. This change may be further complicated by the normal aging processes, work frustrations, family problems, and social pressures.

When you're past middle age, it is not natural to have the same level of reproductive hormones as a young woman.

Menopause and Hormonal Stress

About two to eight years before actual menopause, women may experience menstrual irregularities or lighter or heavier flows. Heavy bleeding or "spotting" should be checked medically to exclude cancer. Fibroids (noncancerous growths in the uterus) are often the cause of heavy bleeding. Fibroids shrink once your periods stop, but women with fibroids tend to be high estrogen producers and often have late menopause.

When your periods stop completely, your estrogen and progesterone levels are low because the body has switched over to hormone levels appropriate for your nonchildbearing years. Your brain and the rest of your body, however, have become accustomed to relatively high levels of estrogen and progesterone.

At menopause, these levels of hormones are no longer available because your ovaries have run out of eggs, so no hormone-secreting follicles can develop. Your hypothalamus and pituitary gland get the message from your blood that your reproductive hormones are low, and they vigorously send out hormonal messengers, hence menopausal women have high levels of FSH and LH. This extra activity by the brain's hormone control center plus the hormonal messengers rushing through the bloodstream are responsible for menopause symptoms. Your brain's control center is "confused" by the lack of response, and it may take a while to reduce the level of stimulating messages.

Although estrogen and progesterone have specific reproductive actions, they travel throughout the bloodstream and tissues, and your body gets used to their presence. In my view, menopausal and postmenopausal women are not deficient in estrogen and progesterone, but many experience hormone withdrawal symptoms while the brain and body are adjusting. Some women don't experience symptoms for a variety of reasons, explained below.

Some scientific studies indicate that the only symptoms clearly associated with menopausal hormone changes are flushing and sweating; dry, thin vaginal skin; possibly palpitations; and loss of bone minerals, which may lead to osteoporosis. Other scientists apparently believe that virtually every physical or mental complaint in middle-age women is caused by lack of estrogen. Estrogen prescription may in fact mask the real cause.

Mainstream medicine establishes that women are estrogen and progesterone deficient at menopause. It has also termed a new syndrome called female androgen deficiency syndrome (FADS), which means that women are also deficient in androstenedione (adrenal hormone) and testosterone (male hormone). As women (and men) age, however, *every* hormone, biochemical, and tissue in the body changes, so according to this classification, all middle-age to elderly people are deficient in hundreds of compounds.

Glands, Organs, and Hormones Involved in Menopausal Changes

The Hypothalamus   The hypothalamus, a part of your brain, monitors and controls hormone levels, aided by the pituitary and thyroid glands. It also regulates appetite, thirst, and body heat.

The Pituitary Gland   The pituitary gland releases FSH to activate estrogen production by the ovaries. This gland also releases LH, which instructs the ovaries to decrease the amount of estrogen production so that the menstrual cycle can occur. At menopause, the ovaries are no longer sufficiently active to respond to the pituitary's hormonal messengers. After menopause, the pituitary gland still produces FSH and LH and high levels of these "messenger" hormones are linked to menopause symptoms such as flushing.

The Ovaries   After menopause, the ovaries begin to shrink; they no longer secrete progesterone and their ability to produce estrogen is markedly reduced.

Progesterone

The word *progesterone* is used to describe the hormone produced naturally by the body; the word *progestin* is used in the United States for synthetic/pharmaceutical versions of the hormone (*progestagen* is the British spelling).

This hormone has no primary function after menopause because its main purpose is to regulate menstruation and pregnancy. At menopause the body abruptly stops producing progesterone. In some women this change is linked to flushing because progestin replacement and progesterone therapy can lower the levels of the pituitary hormones associated with flushing episodes.

Progesterone can be converted to estrogen in the body and can also stimulate an enzyme responsible for converting the body's weaker estrogens to estradiol.

Estrogen

Estrogen is not a single hormone, but a group whose components have similar effects. Estradiol is the main estrogen in your body during menstruation. Estrone is the main estrogen produced by the body in older women. Estriol is the weakest of the body's hormones.

Estrogens are the main hormones responsible for female characteristics. They stimulate cell division of the uterus; increase cervical mucus; affect the growth of breasts, bones, and other tissue; and influence skin, circulation, muscles, fluid balance, nerve function, and behavior.

All these effects are not necessarily beneficial. For instance, high estrogens cause some forms of premenstrual syndrome and are linked to endometriosis, fibrocystic breast disease, and reproductive cancers.

How estrogen actually affects the body depends on enzymes and receptor (receiving) sites throughout the body. Estrogen metabolism also takes place in the liver and the adrenal glands, in fat and muscle tissue, and in the intestines as well as in the reproductive system. Some actions of estrogens are interrupted or influenced by progesterone and other hormones.

No two people produce, absorb, use, convert, or excrete hormones in exactly the same way. In addition, alcohol consumption, age, liver function, intestinal bacteria, body weight, body composition, diet, and environmental factors all affect estrogen activity.

This book proposes that menopause is not a time of estrogen deficiency but of temporary estrogen and progesterone withdrawal as the body adjusts to lower levels. During this transition time the hypothalamus and pituitary are overstimulated. The changing hormonal pattern may be further aggravated by an unhealthy lifestyle, life stresses, and aging.

Why Do Some Women Experience No Menopausal Symptoms?

The degree to which some women experience menopausal symptoms depends on a variety of factors:

- They have favorable genes or good luck.
- They have the ability to handle stress and change relatively easily.
- They have no other major stresses, health problems, work frustrations, or family worries. Or, they have developed good coping skills.
- They have ignored the exaggerated stereotyped information about menopause.
- Their bodies may produce enough estrogen to satisfy biological needs, and the hypothalamus and pituitary are not overloaded.
- The adrenal glands may be very efficient. As well as playing a major role in the ability to cope with stress and change, these glands produce a hormone that is converted to estrogens. This conversion takes place mostly in fat and muscles, so being extremely thin may be a disadvantage during and after menopause. In my clinic I notice an increase in middle-age anorexia, which makes everything worse.
- The decrease in estrogens may occur fairly slowly so that the body and mind have time to adjust.
- They may have had a history of trouble-free menstruation.
- The levels of other hormones and body chemicals may increase the quantity of available estrogens.
- They may be getting a good supply of phytoestrogens (plant estrogens).

Many women still experience symptoms despite their busy and interesting lives. Don't think that it's your own fault if you happen to have menopausal symptoms.

Premature Menopause

Premature menopause is usually defined as the permanent cessation of menstruation before the age of forty-five. Women with premature menopause have blood hormone levels in line with those of older women. Treating premature menopause generally requires the care of a physician because it has many causes:

- Removal of ovaries
- Sometimes hysterectomy alone
- High-dose radiotherapy and some chemotherapy
- Chromosomal disorders such as Turner syndrome
- Metabolic disorders, for example, galactosemia
- Endocrine disorders including ovarian failure, Addison's disease, and thyroiditis
- Immune problems, such as severe fungal infections and mumps
- Autoimmune diseases, such as myasthenia gravis and pernicious anemia
- Prolonged hormone treatment, such as GnRH analogues and occasionally oral contraceptives
- Very poor nutrition, anorexia, extreme overexercising, and trauma

In general, your age at menopause is determined by the number of ovarian follicles you have. Depending on the cause of premature menopause, natural therapies may be helpful and certainly worth trying because they tend to be heart enhancing and cancer preventive.

Women with premature menopause may indeed be estrogen and progesterone deficient. Although I recommend trying natural therapies first, some women choose to have hormone replacement, in which case natural hormone pharmaceuticals are preferable to synthetic hormones.

Young women who have had the ovaries and uterus removed do not always experience menopause symptoms, but they often have serious bone loss, so preventive strategies should be followed as well as periodic bone mineral density checks.

Menopause Is Not a Disease

Menopause is part of the natural aging process; middle-age women's bodies are meant to function on a relatively low level of reproductive hormones. The reality is that a fifty-year-old body is not the same as a twenty-year-old body, and all hormones, cells, tissue, and biochemicals undergo changes. The primary difference between men and women is that the level of reproductive hormones declines abruptly.

Some (predominantly male) doctors still believe that women are tormented because they no longer menstruate and can no longer bear children. They think that our days are filled with despair about losing our looks and our children leaving home. My own unofficial surveys show that middle-age women do not fret about their grown children leaving home. They are too busy being employed full-time, while doing a substantial amount of unpaid work: helping their parents, children, and grandchildren.

SYMPTOMS OF MENOPAUSE

A Norwegian study of 200 women over a ten-year period concluded that hot flashes, sweating, vaginal dryness, and heart palpitations were the only symptoms resulting from menopause. Psychological complaints are secondary; for example, flushing may cause embarrassment and distress, but most studies find no direct association with complaints such as anxiety, depression, or irritability. Menopause, or even hormones generally, cannot be blamed for everything. Keep in mind that the symptoms are generally temporary. The importance of previously existing symptoms, stereotyped beliefs, and social factors was reported in a British study.[1] According to an Australian report, 70 percent of menopause symptoms are stress-related.[2]

A U.S. study carried out by female doctors reported that the so-called menopause syndrome may be more related to personal characteristics than to menopause. These practitioners not only failed to establish a deficiency disease, but also referred to it as a "so-called syndrome." Symptoms reported were related to negative attitudes prior to menopause. The overwhelming majority of women reported relief that their periods had stopped; only 2.7 percent felt regret.

Some pharmaceutical companies circulate questionnaires so that women can evaluate their need for hormone replacement therapy. One such questionnaire is shown in exhibit I.I.

The pharmaceutical company advises that if you score above 15, you probably need hormonal replacement therapy. Ironically, among the groups of students and my own patients to whom I have circulated this questionnaire, those with the highest scores are young male athletes, followed by mothers with young children, and then menopause-age women.

I have gone through much of the HRT promotional material and questionnaires and found a total of fifty-one symptoms supposedly caused by menopause. The stress of changing hormones at menopause is likely to accentuate problems, but exaggerated, incorrect, and negative information is of itself likely to contribute to negative expectations and experiences. When some patients have asked me, "When will I get the menopause?" they look surprised when I reply, "When your periods stop." Many women have been so indoctrinated that menopause is a bad experience that they expect terrible things to happen after they stop menstruating.

Flushing

About 80 percent of women in Western countries experience some degree of flushing. It can be mild heat without any apparent redness; an attractive blush; or red, patchy flushing of the face, neck, and even the chest. Sometimes the heat is followed by a chilly feeling or sweating. The medical description of menopausal flushing and sweating is *vasomotor symptoms*. One interesting aspect of flushing is that placebos (sugar-coated pills without any therapeutic ingredients) work quite well in many women. It's also puzzling that estrogen medications usually help irrespective of the patient's blood estrogen levels, and that some women with very low estrogens don't get any symptoms.

Of course, if your flushing is severe—especially if it keeps you awake at night—you will obviously be anxious, irritable, and tired. No one, however,

Rate each problem	0 (none)	1 (mild)	2 (moderate)	3 (severe)
Lightheadedness				
Headaches				
Irritability				
Depression				
Feelings of being unloved				
Anxiety				
Mood changes				
Hot flashes				
Sleeplessness				
Unusual fatigue				
Backache				
Joint pains				
Muscle pains				
Increased facial hair				
Crawling feelings under the skin				
Decreased libido				
Dry skin: genitals				
Dry skin: arms, legs, body				
Uncomfortable intercourse				
Urinary frequency				
TOTAL SCORE				

EXHIBIT 1.1 **HRT Questionnaire**

has died of flushing, whereas hormone replacement therapy may cause cancer or other serious diseases. And there are nondrug alternatives to help you over this temporary discomfort. It is rare for a woman of fifty-five to still have hot flashes, although a number of older women develop them after they stop taking hormones. In 82 percent of cases, hot flashes disappear in less than a year without any treatment,[3] and in my clinical experience natural therapies can shorten hot flashes to three months or less in the majority of cases.

Possible Causes of Flushing

- Reduced estrogen and progesterone and increased follicle-stimulating hormone and luteinizing hormone are commonly linked to flushing. Women treated with estradiol implants may experience flushing when the implant is "wearing off" despite blood levels of estrogen being relatively high, indicating that the body gets accustomed to a particular level and gets stressed when the level drops. Two women can have the same estrogen level, but only one may experience flushing.
- The changing hormonal pattern may reduce the brain's natural well-being chemicals.
- Menopausal flushing episodes are commonly triggered by emotional stress; in fact, flushing happens to other people, too. Many people get flushed when they're embarrassed or angry and sweat when they're afraid.
- The nervous system (which is linked to hormonal function) may trigger a change in the hypothalamus, which regulates body heat.

Positive Side Effects of Flushing

- The surge in circulation may be linked to the increase in hormonal signals to and from the pituitary gland, which in turn leads to a higher secretion of adrenal hormones. One of these adrenal hormones is converted to estrogen. Therefore, flushing is part of nature's hormone replacement.
- Additional blood flow triggers some beneficial chemical reactions similar to the body's response to exercise.
- The sweating that can follow a flush not only cools you down, but eliminates some of the body's metabolic wastes.

Vaginal Dryness

Between 3 and 15 percent of postmenopausal women suffer from vaginal dryness, the vaginal lining becomes thinner and may itch, there is less genital hair, and the reproductive organs become somewhat smaller. These changes are linked to reduced hormones and the natural aging process. You may have observed that men, too, have noticeable reproductive organ changes. (It's best not to mention, though; I always say that if you don't have something nice to say about someone's appearance, don't say anything.) If natural remedies don't relieve your vaginal problem, get help from a practitioner.

Emotional Problems

A summary of 108 research studies reported the following conclusions:[4]

- Emotional problems do not necessarily increase either during or following menopause.
- Life stresses account for much more of the variation in emotional well-being.
- Having negative preconceptions about the physical and emotional aspects of menopause might lead to greater distress.
- The view that menopause is a deficiency disease is not appropriate for emotional problems and might even reinforce negative preconceptions about middle age.
- If emotional problems are mistakenly attributed to menopause, the problems are masked rather than resolved.
- Ten psychological studies revealed that natural menopause leads to few changes in psychological characteristics with only a decline in introvertedness and reports of hot flashes.[5]

Studies show that negative attitudes toward menopause, lack of social support, poor marital relations, stressful life events, and recent bereavement are also associated with symptoms. Although there is a significant increase in flushing and vaginal dryness, there is no corresponding increase in general physical and psychological complaints. In essence, natural menopause does not have negative emotional or mental health consequences for the majority of healthy, middle-age women.

Social and Economic Factors

A review of ten surveys showed that mainly underprivileged women with low educational levels, low income, and limited employment opportunities suffer most during menopause.[6] Employment apparently protects women of high socioeconomic status but has a detrimental effect on the under-privileged, presumably because the underprivileged have fewer options and the work they obtain is not career- or interest-oriented. Low socioeconomic areas show a higher rate of all mental and physical diseases. One exception is breast cancer, which is markedly higher in the top socioeconomic group, where women are twice as likely to be taking hormone replacement therapy.

Self-Esteem

A common feature of middle-aged women is low self-esteem and poor self-confidence. One of the most endearing female characteristics is that it is rare to find a woman who is comfortable being served first while others are working. Yet, there is a distinction between kindness and servility. Traits such as submissiveness, self-sacrifice, and acceptance of low social, business, or financial status are not as prevalent among young women, who will not tolerate what middle-aged women used to accept: coming home late from work, for example, to cook when her husband and/or teenagers have been sitting around.

Many women have worked hard all their lives and now have higher expectations. If, for example, you've been a diligent administrative assistant for thirty years, you might consider that a promotion is warranted, but for various reasons it doesn't come. When your new twenty-five-year old boss asks you to fetch his coffee, your changing hormones may not be the sole cause of your hot flush.

According to a United Nations report, women make up half the world's population, receive one-tenth of the world's wealth, account for two-thirds of the world's working hours, and own only one-hundredth of the world's property. It's not surprising that we can feel unappreciated and that suppressed frustration may be expressed when we also have to cope with our changing hormones.

"Houseworkitis"

My first case of "houseworkitis," aside from myself, was a woman in her early fifties who wanted something to help her through menopause. Her main symptom was an urge to scream every time she had to do the laundry. We worked out that, with a total of five children, she had washed more than 10,000 loads of laundry over the years. Part of her treatment involved asking someone else in the family to do this chore; there were four other adults in the household.

Another woman told me that she has now refused to do anything at all for her all-male family on Saturdays. She had spent her entire adult life in a full-time job while doing all the household chores every day, year after year. Her family (all adults) now conspicuously avoid her on her "free day." Although most women would understand her, the men in her family are somewhat perplexed.

If you were married at age twenty and had two children, by menopause you've probably prepared over 32,000 meals, ironed more than 20,000 shirts, washed over a million plates, and so on. Don't be surprised if you develop "houseworkitis," but not all women develop this symptom. Sometimes it is suppressed, but outbursts of "vacuumitis" or "dishitis" may pop up unexpectedly. I actually enjoy some domestic jobs—chopping wood, lighting the fire, and making up new recipes—but I always put off the ironing until there is something good on television.

A calm discussion among the adults in the household along the lines of sharing the chores may help. Perhaps you could try swapping jobs. For example, it's better for your bones if you wash the car or do the gardening instead of the ironing or cooking. You'd be healthier if you mowed the lawns and did the gardening and had someone else to do the kitchen work, rather than the other way around. As you will see in chapter 3, it will be beneficial if you and your family discover an interest in cooking, so I've provided a few recipes to get you started. You might even pick up a vegetarian cookbook or be creative and do variations of my recipes.

CULTURE, DIET, AND LIFESTYLE FACTORS

In my clinic, I have noticed that vegetarian women experience less flushing. Apparently, only about 10 percent of Japanese women experience flushing, because vegetarians have a high level of phytoestrogens in their diets.

A comparative study of rural Mayan Indians living in Mexico and rural Greek women[7] revealed that both groups were much more concerned with menstruation and factors related to childbirth than with menopause, which was seen as a life stage free of restrictions and increased freedom. Sexual relationships with their husbands improved because they were relieved from the fear of unwanted pregnancies as well as the menstrual flow, which was considered bothersome. In both societies a good mother is highly regarded and old age is associated with increased power and respect. Older women are also believed to possess special healing skills.

In contrast, Mayan women do not associate menopause with any physical or emotional symptoms. None reported hot flashes, cold sweats, or other symptoms. They report being happy, content, and healthy. Anxiety, negative attitudes, health concerns, and stress for Mayan women are associated with childbearing years. The Greek women experienced flushing and cold sweats but did not perceive that as a disease symptom and did not seek medical intervention. They considered it to be a natural, temporary discomfort.

The striking difference between the two cultures is their diet. The Mayan diet consists of corn, beans, tomatoes, green leafy vegetables, some radishes, squash, sweet potatoes, very little animal protein, and no milk products. Greeks, on the other hand, have a wider variety of foods including wheat, cheese, milk, eggs, plenty of meat, fish, olives, greens, legumes, fruit, and wine. The Mayan diet is much higher in phytoestrogens (plant estrogens); while the Greek diet is much higher in animal protein, which tends to prevent the absorption of phytoestrogens and calcium.

Other Examples of Cultural Differences

When blood estrogen levels of Japanese women were compared with those of women in the United States, after adjusting for weight, it was found that the U.S. women had levels (43 percent higher) linked to higher rates of breast cancer in America.[8] Japanese women also experience a lower rate of bone fractures.

Australian aboriginal women expressed surprise when asked if they experienced menopausal symptoms. In some African tribes, women after menopause graduate from being "bearers of children and drawers of water" to full tribal equality. (I think, however, that the researcher missed the point, as the women should have been treated equally in the first place.)

Some societies apparently reward women for having reached menopause, whereas others seem to punish them, for example, by implying that we should somehow remain forever sexy, young, slender, lively, but servile. Setting impossible tasks is a form of punishment.

In the 1960s a new male species emerged in the United States: aging medical gentlemen, with the peculiar trait of not seeing their own signs of aging and who promoted the bizarre view that women were not "designed" to live beyond childbearing years and therefore all were hormone deficient after menopause. This species spread throughout the Western world, even to underdeveloped countries, and now has an uncontrollable urge to prescribe hormone replacement therapy even to women who are still menstruating. They may tell women that they will lose their femininity, their husbands, and just about everything else if they don't take hormone replacement therapy.

The Positive Side of Menopause

You're already aware of all the symptoms and discomforts of menopause, but think of its benefits:

- Freedom from periods and menstrual problems
- No worries about pregnancy
- Increased knowledge, experience, wisdom, and contentment, which is what aging is supposed to bring, not a futile attempt to recapture youth

- No longer driven by work ambition (perhaps with more time to develop new skills and interests)
- Relief from financial worries. If you haven't made it financially, I hope you have realized that you don't need much to be contented.
- Life not dominated by sex or having dates
- Increased awareness of the need to help other people and improve yourself

The American Psychological Association reported that once estrogen levels decline, your spatial memory skills improve; for example, you become better at tasks such as map reading. Eleanor Hatch, a postmenopausal naturopath, said to me, "I love the way my brain thinks now. It's like I'm able to ponder things as I did when I was a child. I feel sorry for women on HRT because they're robbed of this rejuvenation." One of my patients said, "I enjoy being menopausal because I feel free to say what I like and don't have to conform to other people's expectations."

Aside from population statistics, you know from your family tree that relatively strong, elderly women have always been an important part of society. My own great-grandmother had seventeen children, only two of whom died in childhood. She often had as many as twenty extras for lunch after church on Sundays and was a busy midwife as well. The family was so poor that the children had to take turns at missing school so that they could prevent the farm goats from eating the laundry, which, of course, she did by hand. She was invariably helpful to others, although she never had inside water or a proper stove until she was seventy-five; and she died at seventy-nine, perhaps from the excess luxury! Four of her daughters lived beyond seventy-six years of age; one of her granddaughters taught yoga until she was seventy-nine. When she was eighty-four (weighing 112 pounds) she did my gardening, and she was so strong she could break the trunk of a small tree with her bare hands. None of these women had even heard of estrogen deficiency or hormone replacement therapy.

We all experience menopause differently, depending on our health and circumstances. Why take a risky drug that attempts to put "young hormones" in a middle-age body? Taking HRT tells the body to halt its own production of hormones, so it seems unwise to completely dampen the corrective biological function that already exists. Unless you have a true deficiency disease, such as Addison's or diabetes, you don't need hormonal drugs to keep you alive and well.

You can't avoid the inevitability of aging, but give your body a chance to adjust to menopause the natural way.

CHAPTER TWO

Hormone Replacement Therapy: A Pill of Bad Goods

WHAT IS HORMONE REPLACEMENT THERAPY?

Hormone replacement therapy is a category of pharmaceutical drugs designed and promoted for women who have reached or passed natural menopause or for young women who no longer menstruate due to serious disorders or the surgical removal of the uterus and/or ovaries. The aim of this chapter is to offset the overzealous and often inappropriate promotion of hormone replacement therapy. (Appendix I lists 200 reasons why you should avoid HRT.)

The main hormones used in HRT are estrogen and progestin, usually in combination. *Progestin* is the name given to synthetic progesterone (*progestogen* in the United Kingdom). Some doctors also prescribe testosterone, natural progesterone, and dehydroepiandrosterone (DHEA, an adrenal hormone). Other hormones and hormone-related drugs, such as selective estrogen receptor modulators (SERMs), are also being marketed.

Estrogen Replacement Therapy

Estrogen is the key component of medical replacement therapy. It has therapeutic benefits, notably for reducing menopausal symptoms, and it has valuable secondary functions that include preserving bone and keeping vaginal tissue strong and moist. Both natural and synthetic estrogens can cause or trigger problems, including cancer of the breast and uterus.

There are three basic groups of estrogen medications used in HRT:

1. Estrogens derived from various sources that are chemically similar to the body's natural hormones: estradiol, estrone, and estriol
2. Estrogens produced from pregnant mares' urine (classified as "natural" by the manufacturers and some physicians)
3. Synthetic or semisynthetic (produced in a laboratory but not precisely the same as the body's hormones)

Estrogens (and other hormones) may be prescribed in different forms and must be used as prescribed (for example, a skin cream should not be applied into the vagina):

- Tablets or capsules
- Implants injected into the abdomen or other parts of the body
- Pessaries or rings inserted into the vagina
- Devices inserted into the uterus
- Creams or gels applied externally around or in the vagina or elsewhere
- Patches resembling Band-Aids that adhere to the skin
- Injections
- Lozenges
- Preparations that may be inserted into the nose or under the tongue

Progestin and Progesterone Replacement Therapy

Synthetic progestins are commonly used as part of HRT. Their chemical names include medroxyprogesterone acetate, dydrogesterone, norethisterone, norethindrone, cyproterone acetate, and medrogestone. Although there is no primary need of progesterone after menopause, it is included in HRT prescriptions to offset the "hazards" of estrogen replacement, particularly estrogen's cancer-causing effects on the uterus. Progestins have varying hormonal effects; for example, norethindrone has minor to moderate androgenic properties (producing male characteristics).

Progestins are commonly prescribed in tablet form, although a few physicians use injections. Skin patches and regimes that combine estrogen and progestin are now available.

Natural progesterone is also available in various forms as an internal and external treatment, but there is some doubt about its therapeutic effectiveness and its ability to offset the cancer-causing potential of stronger estrogen drugs. Hence, women using any hormone therapy should be monitored by a medical physician.

Testosterone

Testosterone is the main hormone responsible for male sexuality and characteristics such as facial hair and a deep voice. Women produce tiny quantities. Testosterone may be prescribed to menopausal women as tablets or implants to increase libido (sex drive). It is an anabolic (growth) steroid, and various anabolic hormones are sometimes prescribed to women with osteoporosis.

New Hormone Medications

Selective Estrogen Receptor Modulators (SERMs)   SERMs are claimed to offset postmenopausal bone loss but are not as effective as HRT. They increase the risk of thromboembolism (clots/arterial blockages) but are associated with a significantly reduced risk of breast cancer.

Nonsteroidal Estrogen Receptor Therapeutics (NSERTs)   NSERTs are a potentially safe alternative to current HRT regimens. They have been shown to stimulate rat uteri without increasing proliferation (cell growth).

Other drugs currently being tested include a "designer" (synthetic steroid) agent with estrogenic, progestogenic, and androgenic properties approved in some countries for the prevention of bone loss. It is also suggested for menopausal symptoms for one year after menopause, when the body's estradiol level is presumed to be low.

About forty new types of hormone preparations are currently being developed for women.

HRT REGIMES

Current reasons for prescribing HRT are as follows:

- To reduce menopausal symptoms
- To maintain or slightly increase bone mineral density
- To reduce fractures (if taken for sufficient duration)
- For urinary and genital aging
- To reduce heart disease (lowers cholesterol but increases clots)
- To reduce the incidence and severity of Alzheimer's disease

In the United States, the majority of prescriptions are oral estrogens, which constitute 86 percent of the market. The U.S. market leader of oral estrogens is Premarin, conjugated equine (horse) estrogens (70 percent of the market).[1] There are more than sixty brands of estrogens available, over twenty progestins, and a burgeoning number of combined oral and skin products, plus topical and vaginal medications. For some of the brands there may be five different strengths available. The following are a few examples of types of HRT prescriptions:

- Estrogen for twenty-eight continuous days (usually prescribed when the uterus has been removed)
- Estrogen for twenty-one days, with seven days free each twenty-eight-day cycle
- Continuous estrogen tablets, with added progestin for seven to fourteen days each twenty-eight-day cycle or the progestin every third month only
- Estrogen patches (or tablets) for twenty days, followed by a cycle of progestin for ten to eleven days
- A cycle of fourteen days of estrogen, followed by fourteen days of progestin

- Estrogen for twenty-one days, with progestin for the last ten to fourteen days; no medication during the fourth week
- Estriol vaginal cream (usually prescribed for vaginal dryness and shrinking) applied daily for two to three weeks, then one to two doses per week; discontinued every two to three months to assess if further treatment is necessary

There are many variations in the cyclical regimens and different standards in different countries. Cyclical regimes generally result in monthly bleeding and "spotting," which in my opinion are unnatural effects because the postmenopausal uterus lining is naturally nonactive at this stage of life.

Some practitioners recommend natural estrogen in the form of estriol cream or progesterone in the form of vaginal, skin, or oral micronized preparations. Appropriate trials, however, have not yet been done to prove its effectiveness or safety over the range of therapeutic applications. It is reasonable to assume that natural hormones are "safer" than synthetics.

Increasing numbers of physicians are concerned about the adverse effects of HRT. For example, a U.S. pharmacy journal stated, "The development of new agents with pharmacodynamic profiles similar to that of ERT/HRT but lacking its adverse effects would be greatly beneficial for postmenopausal women."[2]

PROBLEMS ASSOCIATED WITH HRT

Women are typically encouraged to take HRT by their physicians, who cite its benefits—preventing osteoporosis and heart disease—but who minimize its risks. Thus, the rest of the chapter is devoted to a discussion of the problems associated with HRT, in A to Z format.

Adaptation

Some evidence suggests that the body gets used to estrogen medications, which means that the effect wears off in time. For example, one study tested the effect of estradiol implants, estradiol plus testosterone, and a placebo (nontherapeutic pill) on psychological symptoms. Overall, there were no differences between the treatment groups and the placebo group. One group receiving hormones had an initial improvement, but after four months the placebo group improved, whereas the hormone groups did not. Nevertheless, the authors concluded that climacteric depression responds well to HRT.[3]

Addiction

Estrogen implants in particular have been linked to addiction, and medical journals contain reports that women return for more estrogen when their levels are "wearing off" but are still relatively high.[4]

In some women, menopausal symptoms can persist even when estrogens are at high levels. There is also some concern about long-term HRT users with a history of anxiety or depression and possible dependence. Estrogen withdrawal and withdrawal from some types of social drugs have similar symptoms, reinforcing that what makes you feel good is not necessarily good for you. In one three-and-a-half-year HRT trial, withdrawal effects lasted six months. It is better not to get hooked on these potent drugs unless you can be given evidence that your well-being is seriously threatened without them.

Advertising Claims

In the United States, experts from various fields were asked to rate 109 medical advertisements in terms of educational value, scientific rigor, and compliance with government standards. Of these, 40 percent exaggerated a drug's benefits by downplaying its known hazards; 30 percent cited statistics from inconclusive, dissimilar, or poorly designed studies; and 30 percent included misleading graphs or tables. Various studies have found that advertising influences how doctors treat their patients; otherwise, companies would not spend millions on it.

Menopause pamphlets geared toward the general public tend to show women who look about forty years of age. She might indeed be forty, or she might be fifty with the benefit of natural good looks, expert makeup, lighting, and retouched photography. Much of the HRT advertising is based on distortions about menopause, as discussed in chapter 1.

Aging and Longevity

HRT is sometimes promoted as an antiaging agent. Women in the top socioeconomic group, who are more likely to be taking HRT anyway, are expected to live considerably longer than women in lower socioeconomic groups, even without treatment. Poverty and poor education are the major causes of early death, not alleged reproductive hormone deficiency.

Alcohol and Estrogens

Postmenopausal women who are moderate alcohol consumers and who take estrogen replacement therapy further increase their risk of breast cancer because alcohol increases estradiol levels.[5]

Androgens

Androgens are sometimes prescribed as part of hormone replacement therapy. They are, however, associated with a very high incidence of liver abnormalities, including cancer.[6] Growth or male hormones given to older women carry obvious potential side effects.

Animal Cruelty

Premarin, the most widely used HRT drug, is derived from *pregnant mares' urine*. Over 75,000 pregnant mares in the United States and Canada are confined indoors and linked to collecting tubes in tiny stalls for six months at a time, often with limited drinking water so that their urine is more concentrated. This practice spells misery and death for thousands of horses and foals.

Animal Studies

Studies on animals are performed because they have some relevance for humans. Animal studies show that estrogens and progestins are carcinogenic and have been shown to induce cancer not only in target organs such as the mammary glands, uterus, pituitary gland, and ovaries, but also in the liver, lymphoid tissues, adrenal glands, and kidneys. Although epidemiologists may be uncertain of the meaning of these animal studies results, millions of women are being prescribed hormones with a certainty that is not justified by the evidence.[7]

The relevance of any of these findings with respect to humans has not been established. Thus, if the manufacturers and scientific experts are not going to take notice of the animal studies, the animals should not be sacrificed.

Antioxidant Effects of Estrogen Therapy

Estrogen is promoted for its antioxidant effect, notably on (LDL) cholesterol. Cholesterol is found in animal foods and is also produced in the body—which explains why some people have high blood cholesterol levels even though they eat a low fat diet. Cholesterol is divided into two basic types, HDL and LDL: HDL (healthy) stands for high-density lipoprotein, which means that there is a relatively high ratio of protein to fat in each "tiny ball" of cholesterol. LDL (harmful) stands for low-density lipoprotein, which means that each unit contains a relatively low ratio of protein to fat. VLDL (more harmful) stands for very low-density lipoprotein. Both LDL and VLDL are more likely to get deposited in the walls of blood vessels and cause blockages or clots. These harmful fats also cause problems when they oxidize (combine with oxygen in the body), and antioxidants help offset these problems. Progesterone and testosterone, however, do not have this effect.[8] Meanwhile, numerous natural antioxidants such as vitamin E, soy, fruits, and vegetables exist so that no one has to rely on estrogen therapy for this effect.

Anxiety

Reproductive hormones have the capacity to worsen anxiety. In menstruating women, excess estrogens (produced naturally in the body) are related to premenstrual anxiety, irritability, and mood swings. In addition, they are known to stress the pancreas and adrenal glands, which means that they can cause a whole range of nervous symptoms including weakness and shaking.

One patient of mine, for instance, sought a physician's help because she was having serious difficulties with her husband. After a ten-minute consultation, she was diagnosed as being estrogen deficient. The HRT caused her to cry uncontrollably. Her physician told her, "Don't be silly. They make you feel better and if you don't take them you'll end up in hospital with broken bones that won't mend." She was too frightened to come off the hormones, and I could not guarantee her (nor can anyone else) that she wouldn't sustain a fracture some time in the future. I persuaded her to see another physician who immediately took her off HRT and gave her what he described as a safe tranquilizer. Neither physician suggested marriage counseling.

Although HRT improves emotional well-being for a number of women, you should always seek noninvasive treatments first. If one of your parents has died, your husband has left you for another woman, someone in your family is seriously ill, your children are pressing you to be a full-time baby-sitter, or your responsibilities increase, HRT will not resolve issues caused by pressure, stress, guilt, and damaged self-esteem.

Arthritis

Canadian statistics indicate that the incidence of arthritis for current HRT users (who had used hormones for five years or longer) was twice as high as for nonusers.[9] Short-term HRT use (up to five years) was associated with an excess risk of hip osteoarthritis.[10]

Asthma

Postmenopausal hormone therapy increases the risk of asthma.[11] Various medical journals have reported cases of worsened asthma and bronchospasm with HRT, and I've seen similar cases in my clinic.

Back Pain

Swedish researchers report a higher prevalence of back pain in HRT users and speculate that hormonal effects on ligaments and joints are involved.[12] You can verify this finding yourself by examining the joints and tissue of chickens that have been treated with hormones compared with chickens that have been raised naturally.

Biochemical Changes

All hormone medications tend to cause biochemical stress. Protein hormone receptors for estrogen, thyroid, or adrenals are similar; giving one may stimulate the others. HRT estrogen users are more likely to have blood clots, lower bone alkaline phosphatase, increased adrenal stress hormones, decreased defense against infection (lower white blood cell count, proliferation of viruses, more hepatitis), compromised pancreas function, increased antibody levels, and allergies and be less able to deal with carcinogens (due to impaired liver function).[13]

Other reports suggest that little is known about the combined effects of pharmaceutical estrogen, progestins, and testosterone on various blood compounds.[14] Some changes may be good or bad, depending on the status of the patient and other remedies being taken. According to one report, HRT, using conjugated (horse) estrogens and progestin, produces small but sustained changes in acid–base levels.[15]

Bleeding Disorders

Women on HRT have a higher incidence of bleeding disorders, and the cause of bleeding is different compared with nonusers.[16] Abnormal uterine bleeding is not the only uterine problem related to HRT; other problems are listed under endometrial disorders. One paper suggested that an assessment of the uterine cavity and subsequent counseling as to the risk of heavy or prolonged bleeding will be helpful in future management and may improve compliance.[17] One would assume that increased knowledge about bleeding and diagnosis would decrease compliance.

The Cancer Controversy

Breast Cancer   Data based on fifty-one studies on over 160,000 women in twenty-one countries showed that the risk of breast cancer is increased in women using HRT and increases with duration of use. This effect is reduced after cessation of use and largely disappears after about five years.[18] The *Journal of Epidemiology and Biostatistics* states that nearly a hundred epidemiological studies have reported the relationship between HRT use and the risk of female reproductive cancers. The conclusion is that the overall balance between the excess incidence of these cancers and other effects of HRT needs to be evaluated carefully and will require more reliable data than exist at present.[19]

A study of breast biopsies of eighty-six postmenopausal women showed a greater risk from HRT than without HRT and "with estrogen and progestin, breast proliferation was localized to the terminal duct-lobular unit of the breast, which is the site of development of most breast cancers."[20]

Adding a progestin (synthetic progesterone) to the regimen does not reduce the risk of breast cancer. A large U.S. study showed a relative risk of 1.3 for users of estrogen alone and 1.4 for users of estrogen and progestin. The same study also observed a relative risk of 1.7 for current users of at least five years duration among women age sixty to sixty-four. A 70 percent increase in risk for this age group has a large impact on the number of breast cancers produced because of high baseline rates in older women.[21] Experimental synthetic progestins have been shown to increase growth of breast tumor cells, suggesting that progestins are likely to increase the risk.

The association between breast cancer and hormone replacement therapy is still being debated. Some reports now suggest that women who take HRT and subsequently develop breast cancer actually have less invasive cancer and/or recover better. It may be, however, that the cancer is being picked up earlier or that women who take HRT have a healthier lifestyle and may have had less invasive cancers with or without HRT. My clinical experience is that women in upper socioeconomic groups may also take higher-quality natural supplements, which provides better general health and antioxidant status.

Women are consistently told that the risk of breast cancer is very small, whereas the heart protective effect of HRT is greater, but this advice is questionable (see under heart disease below).

One group of U.S. researchers suggests that the risks for the effect of HRT are biased downward due to the way the figures have been analyzed.[22]

This suggestion confirms a number of similar reports about dubious statistics. One U.S. study failed to identify an adverse effect of HRT on breast cancer mortality in patients with stage I–II disease treated with conservative surgery and radiation.[23] No one wants any form of cancer, but there's better survival with early stage breast cancer anyway.

According to the *Journal of Clinical Oncology*, HRT with estradiol-progestin regimens, especially continuously combined, may increase the mammographic (breast tissue) density in a substantial proportion of women.[24] In addition, the *New England Journal of Medicine* reported that since uncertainty remains about the predictive power and potential risks of repeated mammography, this issue is far from clearly resolved.[25]

A report in *Maturitas* suggested that to minimize the risk of any medical-related legal problems later, it may be prudent to ask the patient to sign a statement that she understands the risks and benefits of HRT and recommended that the problem should also be discussed with her partner or another family member or with the patient's oncologist.[26] Would these legal questions arise if there was no risk?

One group dismissed the question of cancer with a statement that the concern was too insignificant to comment on, whereas *The Lancet* reported that "the time course of the breast cancer epidemic in developed countries correlates uncomfortably well with changes in sex-hormone prescribing. Among 121,700 American nurses, deaths from breast cancer increased by 45 percent in women currently taking postmenopausal hormones for five years or more."[27]

Interestingly, menopause and gynecology journals tend to favor HRT for all women, including those with reproductive cancers, whereas cancer journals tend to be more cautious.

Cervical Cancer   One type of cervical cancer is stimulated in response to estradiol, so natural hormone supplementation may not necessarily be superior to synthetic hormones.[28]

Endometrial Carcinoma   Endometrial carcinoma may result from endometriosis of the sigmoid colon following long-term estrogenic treatment.[29] Other cases of cancer have been reported despite progestin in the HRT program.

Warnings about endometrial changes in women on HRT are beginning to appear. One group of researchers concluded that standard criteria for assessing endometrial changes were inappropriate. At least two other groups of researchers have stated that inappropriate criteria present a problem, in addition to diagnostic variations by different laboratory technicians.[30]

Other questions are how much and what type of progestin or progesterone is required to offset the cancer-causing potential of estrogen therapy.

Ovarian Cancer   Ovarian cancer is another risk that needs to be weighed against the benefits of HRT. Long-term estrogen replacement therapy may increase fatal ovarian cancer risk.[31] An analysis of 327 articles revealed that the use of HRT for more than ten years was associated with the greatest risk of ovarian cancer.[32] A reanalysis of four European case control studies found that HRT appeared to promote ovarian cancer.[33]

Other papers suggest a link between HRT and bladder, bronchogenic, pancreatic, and gastric cancers. Despite all the evidence, some researchers are still suggesting that the cancer risk is fictitious and that physicians must be able to counteract the fear of cancer with fact.[34] The argument is that one in eight to twelve women in Western countries may contract breast cancer; one in three over sixty-five years old will have cardiovascular disease, and 30 to 50 percent of postmenopausal women will develop osteoporosis. My counterargument is that heart disease and osteoporotic fractures are mostly problems that occur in the elderly, and there is no clear evidence that HRT will actually prevent these problems in this population.

Cigarette Smoking and HRT

Hormone takers who don't smoke are more at risk of heart attacks than smokers who don't take hormones. The combination of beneficial or negative lifestyle factors and HRT has yet to be determined in regard to osteoporosis and various other health problems.

Commercial Considerations

The estimated cost of the research and development of a single drug for FDA approval is about $300 million (U.S.), according to one pharmaceutical company. Companies have to sell billions of tablets to recoup their costs, which means that newer and safer drugs may never reach the general public.

Another thing to consider is that producing a novel (synthetic) hormone is patentable (that is, someone can own it) and will therefore make more money than marketing a natural, nonpatentable hormone.

Consumer Product Information

Consumer product information on hormone replacement therapy often has significant flaws that impede informed decision making by women. I've managed to find over 200 problems associated with HRT, many of which are supported by scientific or medical reports, so beware if adverse effects are minimized.

Following are some specific examples taken from HRT pamphlets distributed by pharmaceutical companies (these promotional publications are widely circulated and often undated):

- *"With regard to breast cancer, the current consensus of opinion, based on 24 published studies on this subject, suggests that there is no overall increase or decrease in the chances of developing breast cancer."* Because there are over a hundred studies published on this specific topic, it would be relatively easy to select twenty-four that show HRT to be nonharmful.
- *"Side effects are usually mild and settle down after the first couple of months."* This statement may be correct for some women taking HRT, but most of the side effects listed in this chapter are not mild, and the more serious consequences are long term.
- *"Medical studies have found that HRT decreases the risk of cardiovascular disease by about 50 percent."* This statement is simply misleading. Remember that risk does not actually mean the number of people who will develop heart disease. As you will see in the heart disease section below, the only large-scale controlled trial completed so far does not

support HRT. One researcher team now says, "The roller-coaster changes of direction have made decisions by doctors and their patients about the long-term use of HRT extremely difficult and need to be replaced by the stability that only further randomized controlled trials can now provide."[35]

- *"HRT lowers incidence of bowel and rectal cancer."* This statement is not true. A survey of fourteen studies indicates that there is no association between estrogen replacement therapy and colorectal cancer, and long-term randomized control trials would be required to confirm whether any such relationship exists one way or another.[36] Other medical reports confirm that an unbiased study would need to be done because users of HRT tend to have different lifestyles than nonusers.

Costs Related to HRT

Although the cost of HRT may be relatively inexpensive or government subsidized, some researchers suggest that women undergo a full cardiovascular workup to assess the risks and benefits of HRT.[37] This workup is on top of a general physical, gynecological, and cancer risk assessment, plus repeat examinations for breast cancer and assessing the higher level of abnormal uterine bleeding in postmenopausal women who are on HRT. Additional pharmaceuticals may be prescribed to offset the adverse effects of HRT.

One might suggest that to reassure women about their fears of HRT and breast cancer, they should be tested for female hormone levels, testosterone levels, body mass index, waist-to-hip ratio, and mammographic density as well as evaluated alcohol consumption and family history. Other researchers maintain that it is important to identify factors, such as fibrinogen levels, that may predispose women on HRT to thrombotic (clotting) events. HRT users with high bone mineral density have a substantially increased risk of breast cancer, suggesting that all women should have a bone mineral density scan before going on HRT.[38]

Any person placed on a long-term pharmaceutical regimen might be subjected to a wide range of tests on a yearly basis. Can everyone afford this test mania?

Inhibiting the Body's Natural Hormone Production

Hormones are prescribed in pharmacologic doses; that is, they switch off the body's own production. Most hormones that your body produces work on a system known as "negative feedback." Thus, when your body's levels are low, a message is sent to the brain's control center (hypothalamus), which then acts to increase production. Conversely, if you produce enough, the hypothalamus gets the message that it should lower off production. In my clinical experience, some people obviously have difficulty switching back to their natural production once they have taken hormones, which is one reason some physicians sometimes tell women that once they start taking HRT, they have to keep taking it forever. This difficulty in switching on may also explain why women often get flushing when they come off pharmaceutical hormones even though they never experienced symptoms at menopause.

Dementia

HRT is currently being promoted for reducing dementia, Alzheimer's disease, and general brain aging. A group of researchers found that one study showed improved memory when compared with controls (but not when compared with their prestudy status), and the addition of progestins did not oppose the effects. A second study, however, found no positive effects of HRT use on well-being or memory. The researchers stated that the first study may have been related to expectancy effects, because it is difficult to do a double-blind test when women on HRT experience bleeding and reduction of flushing compared with women on placebos.[39]

A large controlled six-year study, known as WHIMS, is currently under way in the United States to test the theory that HRT reduces dementia in women age sixty-five and older. I predict that the study will conclude that blood clotting and other side effects offset any purported brain benefits.

Different Countries

An estimated 20 million women in developed countries are currently using hormone replacement therapy.[40] Manufacturers have a vested interest in protecting and increasing their financial gain in this area. HRT appears to be more of a marketing success rather than a major step forward in human health.

It is difficult to obtain precise figures of HRT usage in various countries, but the figures in table 2.1 have been taken from medical journals and may be reasonably accurate, although they are probably underestimated.

A survey of women in four European countries found that about one-third of perimenopausal and 13 percent of postmenopausal women were currently taking HRT.[41] Women in different Western countries are not that dissimilar. Are some women more cautious, or is there a difference in cost or physician prescribing practices? Are some governments not supportive of HRT because they are worried about extra costs of tests or adverse effects?

In all the surveys I found, high socioeconomic status or education and early or surgical menopause were linked to more frequent HRT use.

Although many researchers maintain that more women would take HRT if they were more knowledgeable, I propose that the opposite is true.

TABLE 2.1 HRT Use Throughout the World	
United States	35–40% between ages 40–60 years (highest usage in the world)
	15% over 65
	7% over 80
Denmark	26.9% (women over 39 years of age)
	Less than 25% used HRT for more than 3 months
	(Sweden is probably higher than Denmark)
United Kingdom	22% have used HRT; 10% classified as long-term users
Norway	19% (45–69 years of age)
Belgium	18.4% (45–65 years of age)
Netherlands	12% (45–60 years of age), average duration 7 months
Italy	8.5% (45–74 years of age)

Different Regimes

More than 100 different HRT estrogen/progestin programs, some of which have not undergone long-term trials, are now available. Millions of women throughout the world have been reassured that the HRT prescribed for them will prevent a range of diseases and that the benefits outweigh the small risk for breast cancer. Have you, though, been given evidence that *your prescription* has been tested according to medical standards, and have you been assessed for *your risk factors*? A ten-minute consultation could not accomplish these criteria.

There are no long-term controlled studies available on many of the popular HRT regimes. It is neither scientific nor sensible to assume that one regime will have the same effect as another.

"Customized" HRT Regimes   Women are often told that their HRT regimes are customized to suit their needs. The reality is that no pharmaceutical hormone can mimic what a healthy body does, that is, fine-tune hormonal levels every minute of every day. Furthermore, if every woman has an individual program, how can anyone know the subtle or long-term benefits and adverse effects? The concept of an individual reproductive hormone program is a myth.

Disease Prevention and HRT

Should healthy women be given a treatment such as HRT when this therapy carries numerous risks, some of which are life-threatening? An editorial in the *Journal of Women's Health* summed it up as follows: "There can be little doubt that HRT is useful for the relief of menopausal symptoms relating to estrogen deficiency. More information, however, is needed about the overall balance of risks and benefits associated with each HRT preparation used for varying durations by women at differing levels of disease risk."[42]

Dissenting Practitioners and Diverse Opinions

A U.S. survey revealed that physicians vary in their beliefs about the benefits and risks of HRT, indicating that it is not as universally favored as promotional material suggests.[43] Some physicians are reluctant to contradict what is deemed to be current medical opinion. There are also some dissenting medical practitioners. For instance, in a letter published in *The Lancet*, a group of doctors wrote: "Not all doctors are reassured by the claims of safety that have encouraged a 'pro-hormone' prescribing philosophy, and this is why DASH (Doctors Against Abuse from Steroid Sex Hormones) has been set up. . . . General practitioners, obstetricians and gynecologists, physicians, psychiatrists, surgeons, oncologists, radiologists, pathologists, and medical scientists have already expressed interest or concern that female steroid hormones are being prescribed to women without respect for their serious side effects. Our aim is to educate doctors about the real dangers of sex hormones, backed up by scientific evidence."[44]

Natural therapy practitioners like myself, who see the short- and long-term side effects of HRT, advocate nonharmful, drug-free methods of treating menopausal symptoms and preventing premature degenerative diseases and bone fractures for the majority of women.

Dosage

One study showed that low-dose estrogen (25 micrograms a day in the form of patches or 0.3 milligrams daily orally) effectively controls postmenopausal symptoms, reduces bone loss, and reduces heart risk.[45] You might wonder why higher doses are often prescribed, because excess estrogen produces a number of serious side effects.

Some specialists suggest an increase or double the dose if HRT does not give the desired therapeutic result. This recommendation assumes that pharmaceutical hormones are the *only* remedy for middle-age women. An increased dose is often continued indefinitely, unless the patient complains of adverse effects. The higher the dose, the more likely you are to get hormone levels well above natural levels, to become addicted, and to suffer adverse effects.

As mentioned in Appendix I, one supplier recommends "the lowest possible dose for the shortest possible time." No pharmaceutical hormone can match the human body for fine-tuning hormone levels and coordinating with other hormones.

Drug Interactions

Pharmaceutical reference texts supply a long list of possible interactions. If you are on any other medication, you should ask your physician about interactions.

Contraindicated drugs for estrogens include:

- Bromocriptine
- Corticosteroids, glucocorticoids
- Corticotropin
- Cyclosporine
- Hepatotoxic medications, especially dantrolene and isoniazid
- Medications associated with pancreatitis, especially Didanosine, Lamividine, or Zalcitabine
- Protease inhibitors, such as ritonavir
- Somatren or Somatropin
- Tamoxifen
- Calcium supplements
- Smoking/tobacco (it is not known whether any increased risks occur with smoking)

Under progestins, interactions include:

- Aminoglutethimide
- Hepatic enzyme medications, such as Carbamazepine, Phenobarbital, Phenytoin, Rifabutin, and Rifampin
- Anytihypertensive agents
- Anticonvulsants
- Anticoagulants
- Hypoglycemic agents
- Theophylines
- Phenothiazines
- Corticosteroids
- ß-adrenergic antagonists
- Tricyclic antidepressants
- Cyclosporin

- Diazepam
- Chlordiazepoxide

Any of the above pharmaceuticals may alter, increase, or decrease the activity of the hormones, or the hormone medication may alter, increase, or decrease the activity of the pharmaceutical.

In addition, other drug interactions have been reported in the scientific literature. Tacrine, a drug used for dementia and Alzheimer's disease, does not break down as readily when used simultaneously with HRT, which means that smaller doses of tacrine may be appropriate.[46]

It is not known how foods, herbs, and natural therapies interact with HRT with the exception of grapefruit juice, which appears to increase the levels of estradiol therapy in the blood.[47]

Duration

My answer to the question, "How long should women take HRT?" is, "Less than one day," whereas some menopause specialists say, "For the rest of their lives."

One report recommends HRT for a five- to ten-year period to improve the bones and protect against fractures and ten years to reduce the risk of heart problems for those in a high-risk group.[48] This same report states that the use of HRT for hot flashes alone is not sufficient reason to take a protracted course and that to persist beyond ten years requires careful counseling. I doubt that taking HRT from age fifty to sixty would do anything to protect fractures when they commonly occur, that is, in very elderly people.

One U.S. study found that of 85 percent of women on HRT, most had been taking it for five years mainly due to physicians' recommendation.[49] My research indicates that other countries have a much shorter duration of use. Only about 8 percent of Dutch women, for example, remain on HRT for more than two years.

The optimum length of treatment is controversial, just as the actual or purported benefits and risks depend on your health and type of HRT prescribed. Is it reasonable to begin treatment at fifty years of age to prevent a condition that may occur twenty or more years later? The average age for diagnosis of breast cancer is sixty-four, heart attack is seventy-four, and hip fracture is seventy-nine years. After sixty-five years of age, you are more likely to die of heart disease than cancer, but no one is sure that HRT actually prevents heart disease anyway. Furthermore, statistics show that older women are extremely reluctant to take HRT; even if it was preventive for heart disease and osteoporosis, would those who might benefit the most (the lowest socioeconomic group and the very elderly) actually take it?

The best advice seems to be the lowest therapeutic dose for the shortest time, or, better still, see a physician or qualified natural therapist for a program that has beneficial rather than life-threatening side effects.

Endometrial Disorders

Abnormal endometrial cell changes found in women on hormone replacement therapy may be difficult to detect in the early stages. This problem is further complicated because different prescriptions (estrogen alone, cyclic estrogen and progestin, and continuous estrogen and progestin) tend to produce different changes.[50]

Women may be advised that any problem will be detected early on, but a number of researchers are still concerned about the subjective aspects of tests, that is, variations among pathologists.

Endometrial Polyps   A Brazilian report indicated that forty-five patients developed irregular bleeding and an increase in endometrial thickness between six months and two years after starting HRT.[51]

Endometriosis   Women who had endometriosis may experience it again when they take HRT. There have also been case reports of newly formed endometriosis linked with HRT, even spreading to the kidneys and diaphragm.[52] A group of U.K. researchers concluded that changes to the lining of the uterus are due to insufficiently offsetting estrogens with progestins.[53]

Environment

At least 20 million women throughout the world are taking HRT, and probably more than 50 million are taking oral contraceptives. In addition, several thousand kilograms of powerful estrogens, such as diethylstilbestrol, zearanol, and estradiol, are given to cattle, sheep, and poultry each year. It has been suggested that the tiny amount excreted in the urine of each individual could amount to a significant quantity overall and may eventually be picked up in our drinking water. It is unknown how this process might interact with various chemicals and pollutants or how it may affect plants, animals, and humans.[54]

Epilepsy

Synthetic estrogen may be associated with an increase in seizure frequency in menopausal women with epilepsy.[55] A number of human and animal studies indicate that estrogen has convulsant properties and progesterone has anticonvulsant properties.

Estrogen and Progesterone Deficiency

Doctors prescribe HRT to correct a deficiency. After menopause, progesterone levels fall to zero or close to it. Along with many other biochemical changes, most hormone levels become lower as we age.

The term *replacement* is misleading. If menopause is a deficiency disease, why do symptoms occur only temporarily in untreated women? Older postmenopausal women do not suffer from hot flashes and night sweats, because their bodies have adjusted to the levels of hormones produced naturally for the nonreproductive years and supported by hormones in foods. Women who take HRT, on the other hand, may have more than five times the amount of estrogen in the bloodstream than they had before menopause, so their symptoms can recur when they stop HRT.

Ethics

Companies and individual researchers do not deliberately set out to harm people, although there have been instances where experiments have been falsified. The problems of exaggerated claims and overzealous promotion have been covered elsewhere in this chapter and certainly exist in natural therapies as well.

Sometimes when drugs and various products are banned in one country because they are considered to do more harm than good, they are subsequently sold to other countries, particularly those that are economically deprived. If a substance isn't safe enough for us, it isn't safe for disadvantaged countries.

False Sense of Security

Some women I have seen in my clinic have been shocked to find that they have severe osteoporosis despite taking HRT for many years. Most did not have a bone mineral density scan to establish their bones' status before taking HRT. Because they were prescribed HRT to protect their bones, they assumed that was all they needed to do. A number of these women did not exercise and had lifestyle and dietary habits that probably offset any potential advantage that HRT may have. Aside from the possibility that HRT might even cause more heart disease than it prevents, it is well accepted that exercise and health-enhancing foods are major factors in preventing cardiovascular problems and that smoking and sedentary lifestyles are major causes.

Fibrocystic Breast Disease

A Japanese study showed that cysts were present and appeared to increase in size in eight of thirty-one patients using estrogen replacement.[56]

Heart Disease, Hormones, and Women

The use of Premarin (modified horse urine estrogen) together with a progestin was studied in 2,763 postmenopausal women with established heart disease (the HERS study). After four years, when compared with the women on a placebo, the incidence of death or nonfatal heart attacks was reported to be statistically the same in both groups.[57]

There were, however, twenty-three more deaths in the HRT group than in the placebo group, and although this number is not considered significant, it nevertheless indicates a possible unfavorable trend and is not an endorsement for HRT as a heart protectant. In the group receiving HRT, there were three times more clotting incidences and 36 percent higher gallbladder disease than in the group receiving a placebo. Even though horse estrogen may lower LDL cholesterol levels, it is important to remember that cholesterol is only one factor and may be offset by increased clotting. In the HRT group there were more heart attacks in year 1 of the study and fewer in years 4 and 5. You may or may not be placated knowing that HRT causes more deaths in the first year of taking it than in subsequent years.

In the United States, more educated, affluent women, who are also leaner and have more favorable heart disease risk factors before treatment, are those more apt to be treated with HRT. Compliant women who stay on estrogen are the minority of women for whom it is prescribed; compliant women differ in other ways from less compliant women. More frequent visits to the physician may prompt other evaluations and interventions that reduce the risk of heart disease. The Women's Health Initiative, a randomized controlled trial of estrogen plus progestin versus placebo in more than 26,000 women, is still in the recruitment phase and is expected to continue until at least 2006. Pending the results of these and other trials, benefit–risk rates can only be estimated. Also, the optimal dose and regimen for hormone replacement therapy are unknown, as is the best time to start or stop treatment. Meanwhile, the physician and patient together need to define each individual patient's risks and preferences in the context of the available evidence.[58]

It is highly probable that a new range of HRT drugs will be on the market shortly, but these new drugs may not be comparable to older ones in regard to total benefits and negative side effects.

One study shows that Tibolone (a new hormone remedy that alleviates flushing and prevents bone loss without causing monthly bleeds) actually reduces the good cholesterol. This finding is a potentially adverse reaction.[59]

The common opinion of the medical profession is that estrogens have heart protective effects, but because most women are prescribed progestins along with estrogen replacement the question remains, Do progestins off-set this protection? The answer is not clear and depends on the particular estrogen and progestin being prescribed and the health status of the women.

Is there any advantage in lowering cholesterol but increasing clots and triglycerides? (One HRT study showed a 25 percent increase in triglyc-erides.) Is there any advantage in using HRT to lower cholesterol if you have normal levels? Cholesterol has a number of important functions in the body, and low levels are linked to depression and suicide.

In the Framingham Heart Study, postmenopausal estrogen users had 30 percent more heart disease and twice as much cerebrovascular disease than nonusers.

Women are told there is a dramatic increase in heart disease during menopause and they have the same risk of heart attacks and complications as men. These statements however, are simply not true (see table 2.2).

Women are typically told that after menopause they have the same (or more) heart problems and heart attacks than men because postmenopausal women have low estrogen levels and need HRT. In fact, only when women are over eighty-five years of age do they begin to have the level of heart attacks even approaching that of men; surely this rate is due to old age, rather than lack of estrogens. When any practitioner quotes statistics to entice patients to take any remedy, the figures should be correct.

Whenever you are looking at statistics, remember that women who take HRT are in better health to begin with compared with women who don't take hormone replacement. In my opinion, it would seem reasonable to take steps to see if you are at risk of a heart attack before taking so-called pre-ventive pharmaceutical medication that can cause many serious side effects. For example, do you have high LDL cholesterol, high homocysteine, or a family history of heart problems? Could you achieve the desired result through natural supplements, diet, and lifestyle adjustments? One U.S. study concluded that "cardiorespiratory fitness is an important independent deter-minant of blood lipid and fibrinogen levels in nonsmoking postmenopausal women, with or without HRT."[60] Keeping fit is clearly necessary.

TABLE 2.2 **Causes of Death (per 100,000)**

	Males	Females
45–54 years		
Ischemic heart disease	62.5	13.8
Acute heart attack	35.4	9.2
55–64 years		
Ischemic heart disease	203.7	60.6
Acute heart attack	117.8	37.6
65–74 years		
Ischemic heart disease	636.0	262.9
Acute heart attack	388.0	165.8
75–84 years		
Ischemic heart disease	1,747.7	1,039.3
Acute heart attack	1,051.8	654.2
Over 85 years		
Ischemic heart disease	4,150.0	3,559.6
Acute heart attack	2,377.1	1,965.8

Source: Australian Bureau of Statistics 1998 (Catalog No. 3303.3). Americans have similar diets and lifestyles as Australians, so there is no reason to suppose that the statistics are much different in the United States; the figures, however, will be somewhat higher for both men and women because Australians (along with at least fifteen other countries) have a longer life span and better health status than Americans.

Note: The incidence of heart disease does not rise dramatically in women following menopause.

One researcher warns that a sixty- to seventy-year-old woman with heart disease who chooses HRT for other reasons, such as osteoporosis, should be on a low-dose estrogen, should take anticoagulant therapy such as aspirin, and should have a complete heart workup before starting on HRT.[61] Meanwhile, there are over thirty adverse effects and problems associated with aspirin, including an increase in osteoporosis, so aspirin might cause more problems than it solves.

History and Hormones

Historical evidence does not support the use of reproductive hormonal drugs. Decades after diethylstilbestrol was prescribed to pregnant women, it was linked to urinary/reproductive cancers and abnormalities in their children. Pituitary hormone injections used for infertility are now being linked to Creutzfeldt-Jakob disease (the human equivalent of mad cow disease). Negative effects of hormone therapy are long term. Provera, for example, listed "no untoward side effects" in 1984, but by 1999, there were thirty-two listed cautions and adverse effects.

Hostility

Women on estrogen therapy may became less outwardly aggressive but more inwardly hostile. The male hormone, testosterone, is sometimes used as part of HRT for women with low sexual desire, but it may increase anger. Counseling may be more effective than prescribing male hormones for the total well-being of women.

Hypertension

Women with normal blood pressure are at low risk of developing problems from HRT, but there is not sufficient evidence on the effect of HRT in women with high blood pressure.[62] HRT use is not recommended with severe uncontrolled hypertension. I have seen a number of women whose blood pressure was normal but increased within a short time of starting HRT.

Immune System

Immune subsets, such as natural killer cells, were shown to be affected by HRT.[63] Natural killer cells function as anticancer and antimicrobial sentries, so anything that reduces them is not beneficial. Estrogens, however, also stimulate some of the cells that destroy unwanted compounds in the body. The overall effect is not clear, and these changes may be stressful because the body aims for balance. Natural menopause, as distinct from aging, has not been associated with any specific change or defect in the immune system.

Inappropriate Prescribing of HRT

Some women are prescribed HRT for various symptoms even though they are still menstruating normally. One study showed that bladder weakness and flushing in these younger women is not relieved by HRT.[64] A researcher warns that women who take HRT while still menstruating should not assume that it is a reliable contraceptive.[65] Another researcher states that the majority of women on HRT have no signs or symptoms of the diseases for which prevention is being recommended.[66]

One of my patients had recently visited a physician for a problem not linked to menopause, and the doctor strongly urged her to take HRT. When she refused the prescription, he told her she was in denial but did not deal with her current problem, nocturia (nighttime urinating), which cleared with an herbal formula within a week.

Lack of Informed Decision Making

There are major dissimilarities between information available to the medical community and that prepared for the general public. Some of this information may be fundamental for a woman deciding whether or not to take HRT.

For instance, an article states that "postmenopausal diabetic women should be considered for HRT provided the physician is aware of the possible problems and the patient is sufficiently counselled to make an informed decision."[67] These considerations would depend on the bias of the physician, whether the physician had time to assess all the published material and then assess all the risk factors of the individual patient, whether anyone had time to go over all the data with the patient, and whether all the necessary tests had been done.

Mammographic Density and Breast Pain Increased

Both breast tissue density and pain increased in women receiving HRT.[68] An Australian study suggested that in countries where HRT use is widespread, the reduction in sensitivity with HRT may undermine the capacity of population-based mammographic screening programs to realize their potential mortality benefit; in other words, the test is not reliable for HRT users.[69]

Increased breast tissue density associated with HRT has been confirmed in at least seven medical reports, and my clinical observation is that some women complain of breast tenderness that they had not experienced prior to taking HRT. Other women say that their breasts are sore or more sensitive for weeks after mammography.

Medical Trials

Double-blind placebo controlled studies are the typical medical method of establishing the effectiveness and safety of pharmaceuticals. There are a number of problems with these studies.

- These trials are invariably supported by pharmaceutical companies.
- Most are relatively short-term, whereas hormone therapy is linked to both long-term benefits and long-term adverse effects.
- If trials are long term, are the currently healthy people advised if there is a change in the risk factors of the drug being tested so that they can decide whether or not to continue?
- How many trials are not published?
- How can such a study be double blind? Most women taking a potent hormone are likely to know within a few days if they are on the hormone or a sugar pill because no one will deny, for example, that HRT is effective at reducing hot flashes and that bleeding will certainly indicate that they're on the drug.
- Women undergoing trials have contact with health professionals, which are usually "sympathetic" interviews (reinforcement of the notion that they are helping others by participating), and these interviews may encourage positive thinking, thereby reducing symptoms such as flushing.
- Some women also chew and taste the tablet and compare notes with their friends. Sometimes the tablets are marked in such a way that the actual remedy is identifiable so the women know if they are taking the remedy or the placebo. Others take various natural therapy

remedies that may either increase or lower the effectiveness of the drug being tested.

- Often the results of the trials can be interpreted differently. For example, one well-known U.S. trial indicated that after three years, HRT lipid profiles improved. Subsequently, this "segment" of information was circulated to the public, implying that HRT prevented heart disease when in fact there was a trend toward increased cardiac disease in the estrogen groups.[70] In other words, the women may have had lower LDL cholesterol or other positive blood readings but they had worsening heart problems. (See the discussion on heart disease, hormones, and women, on page 42.)

- The short-term effects of most HRT regimes on blood lipids are well known, but it has been suggested that these effects vanish in time, presumably because the body adapts to most hormones. It is not known if and how long it might take for the body's lipids to become insensitive to HRT.

- Since the 1970s, there have been hundreds of trials using HRT, but most specialists are still calling for more realistic or relevant evidence.

One study reported that oral micronized progesterone was an attractive means of supplementation in postmenopausal HRT without any liver-related side effects,[71] but this four-month study did not consider whether or not this progesterone offset the harmful effects of estrogen on the uterus. Of course, one trial cannot study everything, but the human body does hundreds of things simultaneously, so examining one aspect is interesting but not necessarily relevant overall.

Some large-scale medical trials are under way comparing HRT with a low-fat diet and with vitamin D and calcium supplementation in regard to breast cancer, heart disease, and osteoporosis. I argue that this diet is not necessarily healthy. For example:

- Essential fatty acids are needed for health; some types of fats such as virgin olive oil and walnuts appear to reduce heart disease and lower LDL cholesterol.

- Some high-fat foods, such as soy, are considered to be protective against breast cancer.
- Fish oil helps calcium metabolism.
- Essential fatty acids are needed in the body for carotenoid uptake. Carotenoids are among nature's most powerful antioxidants. Lutein, for example, is a carotenoid that maintains the integrity of the retina (eye). Antioxidants help break down some cancer-causing compounds.
- A low-fat diet might mean weight loss. In menopausal women, weight loss invariably means that calcium pours out of the bones (covered in chapter 6).

I argue further that calcium and vitamin D are not the only nutrients necessary for bone health, and they have already been tested extensively with marginal or debatable success. Vitamin D is not necessarily good for everyone, and a wide spectrum of nutrients is required.

If a comparison is being made between a pharmaceutical and a natural therapies program, the latter needs to be clearly healthy; on the other hand, the results may be further confused if the women on the program consume phytoestrogens or take their own supplements.

Menopause Clinics

Menopause clinics tend to be strongly HRT-oriented rather than encouraging women to attain the information, skills, and resources to help themselves and be in control. Germaine Greer has described how some European women volunteer their services and even raise funds to help establish menopause clinics, which are basically outlets for the distribution of replacement hormones.[72] Such women are described as the perfect experimental guinea pigs because they not only feed themselves and keep their cages clean, but pay for their medication, recruit further experimental subjects, and help promote the products.

My experience is that some clinics test natural therapies but often in such low doses (for instance, 40 milligrams isoflavones daily) or they test products with the slightest results (wild yam cream is a good example).

Mood Swings

A Swedish study confirmed that there were no differences between HRT users and nonusers regarding negative mood and sexual desire.[73] Although most women with menopausal symptoms report that they feel better on HRT, a number of studies show that HRT does not improve mood by affecting the brain directly. Everyone, however, feels happier when symptoms are alleviated.

Muscle Weakness

Many women complain that they put on weight if they take HRT. I have observed a number of cases of fluid retention from HRT. One study showed that oral estrogen therapy increases fat mass while reducing lean body mass.[74] Another study showed that HRT resulted in a progressive loss of fitness. This study confirms my observations as a yoga teacher for over twenty-five years: women on HRT have weak muscles, and even a mild muscle injury takes a long time to heal.

An Israeli study showed that HRT does not change weight or fat accumulation, but it minimizes the shift from female to male distribution.[75] Thus, HRT tends to keep the fat in the lower part of the body compared with the upper part.

"Natural" HRT

Women are frequently told that HRT simply puts natural hormones back into their bodies. As explained earlier in this chapter, many HRT pharmaceuticals are synthetic. Estrone is the main estrogen produced in the body by postmenopausal women, yet there are remarkably few estrone drugs.

Also, in nearly every instance, synthetic or semisynthetic hormones have a much longer life than natural hormones. For example, Equilenin (in Premarin) has pronounced hepatic effects and a prolonged half-life,[76] which means that the liver is affected and that a particular estrogenic metabolite stays in the body for a longer period than does natural estrogens.

Hormone drugs produce marked fluctuations in the human body. When drug hormones are taken, there is usually a high initial increase within the body. For instance, one study of women with endometrial cancer showed that four hours after an estradiol tablet was taken, there were blood levels of estrogen above naturally occurring levels despite it being combined with progestin.[77] In these women with endometrial cancer, a hysterectomy was necessary, another less publicized risk of HRT.

Natural progesterone is currently being promoted by some physicians and natural therapists as the best hormone for menopausal women. Yet, from a natural point of view the only organ that actually needs progesterone is the uterus.[78] The uterus, however, no longer has a function in postmenopausal women.

Noncompliance

A U.S. survey found that after one year, 54.4 percent of women were no longer taking HRT. The researchers concluded that increased efforts to improve long-term compliance are urgently needed.[79] Numerous researchers plaintively ask why there is such poor compliance on HRT. My answer is that women may be enticed into starting HRT but abandon it for good reasons. We may or may not understand pharmacology, but we know when something doesn't suit our bodies.

Osteoporosis and HRT

HRT (and birth control pills) causes tiny blood clots that impair the blood supply needed for trabecular bone. If a woman takes HRT for five years after menopause and then discontinues it, her bone loss in ten years remains the same as nonusers.[80] In the United States, women over seventy-five who had taken long-term estrogen therapy and those who had not, had marginal difference in bone mineral density levels.[81] Discontinuation of HRT therapy is followed by immediate resumption of bone loss at a rate similar to that in untreated women.[82] Bone mineral density ten years after stopping is similar to that in women who have never taken menopausal hormones.

Other researchers report that vertebral fracture rates are decreased by about 40 percent and that hip fractures are also decreased. A study on younger women, however, may not apply to the elderly. At least half of all hip fractures occur in women after age eighty.

A British study suggests that taking hormone medication is associated with a reduction in essential bone nutrients and reduced bone formation. International incidence data show that fractures among women aged thirty-five to sixty-five years have increased dramatically in hormone prescribing countries.[83]

The first prospective trial confirmed a beneficial effect of HRT on prevention of peripheral fractures in young nonosteoporotic postmenopausal women.[84] Curiously, this trial did not test fracture risk for older women. In addition, it did not compare HRT with something more effective than low-dose vitamin D.

One researcher writes that "the importance of the menopause to the problems of osteoporosis has been overemphasized." Other factors are important in determining fracture risk and logical preventive strategies should be developed.[85]

I could not find any clear minimum effective dosage, type of hormone, timing, and duration of HRT for fracture prevention. Questions about long-term safety and quality of life still remain.

Other Hormones Given to Menopausal and Postmenopausal Women

Depo-Provera   Although this pharmaceutical is not recommended for menopause, it is sometimes prescribed by medical practitioners for this purpose. In other words, drugs are not always used according to the official indications. A study showed that Depo-Provera (medroxyprogesterone acetate) significantly reduced bone density in premenopausal women.[86] Depo-Provera is an injected, long-lasting contraceptive that has been linked to breast cancer over a number of years.[87] Just one injection seems to influence cancer growth for the next five years. (Provera, the tablet form, is not as strong as Depo-Provera.)

Testosterone   Some HRT regimes include testosterone mainly for increasing libido, even though this therapy is underresearched as a female treatment. Testosterone implants have been fairly widely used, and patches are now available. An Australian study of 201 women found no evidence of a role for testosterone in female sexual functioning.[88] Despite this, testosterone is also prescibed for female depression.

Growth Hormone   Growth hormone is now being suggested as a treatment for female osteoporosis.

Dehydroepiandrosterone (DHEA)   This adrenal hormone has been shown to reduce flushing and psychological symptoms associated with menopause; it also increases testosterone levels.[89] Women of all ages are obtaining and using DHEA without any practitioner supervision, on the basis of promotional material that promises to restore youthfulness and vitality. Inappropriate use, however, can interfere with normal hormone metabolism and may increase cancer risk. DHEA is extensively promoted as an antiaging hormone and is available over-the-counter, by mail, and through the Internet. In Australia it is illegal for anyone other than a medical practitioner to prescribe hormones, but anyone, for example, can order DHEA, progesterone, etc. from the United States. Some people may think more is better. Inappropriate use of all hormones is potentially dangerous because when you take them the body responds by reducing its own production. This is called negative feedback. Steroidal hormones, as a group, generally encourage cell growth in specific tissues of the body, which explains why they are often linked to cancer. That's why most countries do not permit over the counter sale of hormones, natural or otherwise, and people need to be warned about self-treating with them.

Melatonin and Pregnenolone   Melatonin and pregnenolone are being promoted as natural hormones that restore youth and vitality. Although these natural hormones may have fewer side effects than synthetic hormones, they are potent medicines that need to be used with caution. If you thoroughly research the medical and scientific journals, you will find many questions and problems in relation to these hormones. You need to know:

- Are they free from impurities?
- Do they come from animals or plants, or are they laboratory produced?
- Is the product government approved and regulated?
- Are the hormones actually absorbed into the body, and do they reach the target tissue?
- Will they dampen the body's own production of those particular hormones?
- What is the optimal dose and duration?
- Do they interfere with other drugs, hormones, or natural substances?
- Who should take them?
- What are the side effects?
- Have properly controlled long-term studies been done to assess their benefits?

Panic Disorder

Estrogen-induced panic disorder, which is reversed when estrogen is discontinued, has been reported.[90] Panic disorder may be widely unrecognized, and women may be prescribed antianxiety medications without considering that hormone therapy is the cause.

Polypharmacy

Medical specialists used to prescribe estrogen by itself until it was discovered that this practice led to endometrial (uterine) cancer. Then it was discovered that progestins (synthetic progesterones) offset this particular harmful effect. The trouble with progestins is that they, too, have a long list of adverse effects including fluid retention.

While writing this segment, I saw a healthy fifty-four-year-old businesswoman who had gone for a checkup twelve months earlier, and although nothing was medically wrong (aside from a small soft cyst at the back of her neck), her doctor persuaded her to take HRT on the grounds that it would protect her heart and give her a longer, healthier life. Because she still had her uterus, she was prescribed not only a synthetic estrogen but progestin to offset the side effects of estrogen. Within six months, she experienced swelling of the hands and feet, and the cyst increased markedly in size. She returned to her doctor who told her (incorrectly) that once HRT has been started it cannot be discontinued, and he then prescribed a diuretic for the fluid, telling her that it didn't have any adverse effects (also incorrect) and advising that the cyst should be removed surgically. If she continues with his advice, it is possible that within the next six months she could have an adverse reaction to the diuretic, be prescribed yet another pharmaceutical, and go through surgery, as well!

"Preventive" HRT

A survey of over 2,000 American menopausal and postmenopausal women who were long-term users and expected lifetime users of HRT showed that they were not more likely to be using HRT if they had osteoporosis, heart disease, or risk factors for heart disease.[91]

Aside from the reality that HRT may not actually prevent heart disease or osteoporotic fractures in the elderly, how can a drug be truly preventive when it alleviates one problem such as menopausal flushing but causes serious diseases?

Breast cancer risk is associated with estrogen combined with testosterone-derived progestins and appeared especially pronounced with continuously combined regimens.[92] I do not doubt that estrogen reduces cholesterol levels, but the same HRT regimen increases blood clots and triglycerides. One study reported a 25 percent increase in triglycerides.[93]

Progesterone and Progestins

Progestins (Synthetic Progesterone)   Progestins are somewhat different chemically from natural progesterone, and they also last longer in the body and have different effects. Progestins are also somewhat different from one another.[94] Thus, if you have decided to take HRT because of a particular risk factor, you need to ask if the type of progestin in your prescription was the same used in the trial showing a benefit for that factor. For instance, a few studies have shown that one type of progestin as part of HRT lowers the good cholesterol, which is not beneficial. A number of reports suggest that progestins reduced the beneficial effect of estrogens on cholesterol and may increase triglycerides.

Synthetic progestins are not readily broken down; therefore, they have the capacity to offset some undesirable aspects of estrogen therapy, but their prolonged or unusual actions also lead to adverse effects. None of the synthetic progestins has effects identical to natural progesterone, simply because they are different chemically and are not well tolerated by a large proportion of women.

The question remains, Does a low level of progestin or progesterone offset the uterine disadvantages of estrogen? A study using 2.5 milligrams medroxyprogesterone was reported as possibly inadequate as part of continuous combined HRT with respect to offsetting endometrial carcinoma.[95] In other words, if the dose is low enough to prevent bleeding, it may not be cancer protective to the uterus.

Women report adverse symptoms similar to premenstrual syndrome while taking cyclical progestin as part of HRT.[96]

Natural Progesterone A study concluded that medroxyprogesterone acetate (a progestin) reverses the effect of long-term estrogen therapy with respect to exercise-induced myocardial ischemia (lack of oxygen to the heart) but that vaginal progesterone at 90 milligrams every other day did not have this detrimental effect.[97]

Oral micronized progesterone was shown not to have any liver-related side effects after four months of treatment.[98] Four months of treatment is unrealistic, however, given that physicians commonly advise women to stay on HRT for upward of five years; further, other side effects were not studied.

Various forms of natural progesterone are now available, and they have biological effects in the body. A disadvantage of these natural hormones is that they are relatively new and have not been thoroughly studied. My experience is that natural progesterone cream is effective for menopausal symptoms in some women and is certainly worth trying because it seems to have remarkably few short-term effects. A study showed that it improved flushing in 83 percent of women, compared with 19 percent on placebo.[99]

The following questions remain in respect of all forms of natural progesterone:

- Is progesterone effective for reducing heart disease and improving memory?
- Does natural progesterone cream improve bone mineral density, or is density improved by the nutritional supplements in the program?
- Does progesterone have to be prescribed with estrogen?
- What is the optimal dosage when progesterone is prescribed alone or in conjunction with estrogen?
- What is the optimal duration of progesterone use?
- What is the most effective method—oral, skin, or vaginal—of prescribing progesterone?
- Does progesterone contribute to cancer?
- Is progesterone appropriate for all women? Progesterone is essentially a reproductive hormone and the basic function of reproductive hormones is to stimulate reproductive tissues. Is this stimulation necessary or wise for postmenopausal women?

Progesterone, like any other hormone, can have adverse effects. In the few trials that have been conducted, oral micronized progesterone caused headaches and drowsiness even after short-term treatment. Other potential problems include all those listed for synthetic progestins, although the side effects might occur only after long-term use. There are no studies on long-term use. Although progestins (synthetic progesterones) are somewhat different chemically to natural progesterone, it is possible that over many years the natural form of the hormone will produce side effects similar to those listed for the synthetic form.

It is generally agreed that micronized oral progesterone has physiological effects in the body; it helps some women with menopausal symptoms and may stimulate new bone formation.

The dosages and effects of skin and vaginal products are less clear. One research group states that the only practical nonoral means to prescribe progesterone is vaginally. Another study showed that 100 milligrams oral or vaginal progesterone was not sufficient to offset the uterine stimulatory effects of 1.5 milligrams estradiol gel.[100]

Some U.S. physicians are using natural progesterone for osteoporosis and report 2 to 23 percent increase in bone mineral density in three years.[101] I have seen similar results in women using supplements and exercise, however, and I have seen some cases where natural progesterone has not been successful. As discussed in chapter 6, the first controlled scientific trial showed that in a one-year program progesterone cream was no different than placebo. Others report that natural progesterone protects against breast and endometrial cancer, but this has not been proven.

It is probably true that menopausal women are progesterone deficient compared with younger women, but because postmenopausal women have survived successfully into old age for many thousands of years without this hormone, it is not a true deficiency.

The main point is that all hormones—even those produced in your body—are potent compounds, which is why they can cause so many problems.

Psychological Symptoms

Women who report emotional problems to their physicians are sometimes prescribed hormone replacement therapy. Unless severe flushing and sweats cause distress or prevent sleep, however, the majority of psychological symptoms are not convincingly linked to the endocrine changes of menopause.[102] A number of reports indicate that psychological benefits of HRT are more likely to be a result of alleviation of flushing than a direct effect of HRT.[103] Emotional well-being is more related to current health status and psychosocial and lifestyle variables than endocrine changes.[104]

Women who intend to go on HRT report significantly lower self-esteem, higher levels of depressed mood, anxiety, and negative attitudes to menopause. They also expressed a stronger reliance on their doctor's ability to control their menopause experience than on their own ability. These results suggest that some women might be seeking HRT at menopause to help alleviate preexisting emotional difficulties.[105]

Despite these reports, many of the women I see who are on HRT report that they feel more stable emotionally, and my assessment is that HRT seems to give this benefit more to women who are under work, financial, or family pressures. Helping to cope or solve problems may be better treated with counseling than with hormones.

Risks Versus Benefits

Even those who actively promote HRT agree that practitioners should counsel women regarding the risks and benefits. In twenty years, I have not seen one woman who has been given a list of all the potential risks, over 200 or more! Furthermore, it's not always possible to evaluate your risks and benefits in a ten-minute consultation. A number of patients tell me that they haven't even finished discussing their symptoms before a physician is already writing out the prescription.

It is possible that HRT promoters deliberately focus on breast cancer versus heart disease to divert attention away from the numerous other side effects. Most women are surprised to learn about the long list of real and potential problems associated with HRT. Women are also surprised to learn that the purported benefits are not fully supported in scientific and medical studies and reports.

If you are ill, you may be willing to accept a substantial risk of side effects to get potential benefits of a drug, but menopause symptoms rarely constitute a disease. Women on HRT are likely to be exposed to an ever-increasing barrage of tests and scans that also carry at least a small element of risk, such as increased radiation exposure from repeated mammograms.

If you choose not to take HRT, however, you can be confident that there is much support for your choice.

Safer Hormones Are Not Always Prescribed

It has been suggested that estradiol and estrone are likely to trigger cancer, whereas estriol—an estrogen that is produced less abundantly in the body—

is possibly anticarcinogenic. Earlier papers referred to estriol as the forgotten hormone. Estriol is available in tablet form and as a vaginal product.

Japanese researchers found that 2 milligrams daily of oral estriol appeared to be safe and effective in relieving symptoms of menopausal women. . . . Overall, estriol may serve as a good choice for hormone replacement therapy to protect against other climacteric symptoms in postmenopausal women who do not need medication for osteoporosis or coronary artery disease.[106]

Natural progesterone is safer than synthetic progestins, but because it may not be strong enough to balance potent estrogen replacement hormones, it is not commonly prescribed as part of HRT.

Sex   You've probably heard that HRT will improve your sex life, but a decrease in sexual activity is more likely due to age and psychosocial factors. This is covered in chapter 11 in more detail.

Systemic Lupus Erythematosus (SLE)   The risk of systemic lupus erythematosus (SLE) is increased with increasing use of estrogens, according to a survey that followed over 69,000 women for fourteen years.[107] There is some debate regarding the prescription of HRT to women who already have this disease, but again, the debaters in this field tend to look at lupus versus the promoted benefits rather than SLE plus the potential adverse effects of HRT.

Statistics   Incorrect "impressions" are sometimes given inadvertently or purposely. For instance, Australian women aged sixty-five to seventy-four have a 6 percent relative risk of heart disease. This figure translates to 6 of every 100 women within that age group running the risk of heart problems. A 50 percent reduction in the number of women at risk represents a gain of 3 women per 100, rather than the commonly perceived 50 per 100. As explained in this chapter under the heading "Heart Disease, Hormones, and Women," risk is not the same as actual; one trial lowered LDL cholesterol, thereby theoretically reducing the risk of heart attacks, but more women in the trial actually had a heart attack.

The explanation is that all the risk factors have not been considered. If your triglycerides go up or you get a blood clot, your cholesterol levels may or may not be relevant. Furthermore, lowering cholesterol may reduce the risk of heart attacks by a certain percentage, but it is probably equally irrelevant if you have normal LDL cholesterol.

As mentioned in the discussion of heart disease, hormones, and women (see page 42), incorrect information is sometimes given in regard to the number of people who have particular diseases. Incorrect figures are also published in regard to osteoporosis.

The results of trials can be interpreted differently by different experts, but one should always be alert to the differences between "risk" and "incidence" (actual). Also be alert to the source of the figures; unfortunately, the sources are often incorrect.

One report indicates that women who had ever used HRT had a 30 percent lesser probability of dying of any cause and a 40 percent lower probability of dying from colon cancer specifically during the follow-up period.[108] Is it likely that these same women might have better survival times had they not used HRT? All the surveys I have seen show that women in the top socioeconomic group have a much better health outcome to begin with. You'd probably be better off without HRT.

Stroke

Women are told that HRT reduces the risk of stroke. Again, be aware that risk is not the same as incidence. A U.S. study actually showed no evidence that HRT prevents stroke in older women.[109] The largest U.S. study (of nurses) reported no difference in stroke incidence between users and nonusers.[110] A Danish study and a British study also came to the same conclusion.

Suicide and Mental Illness

Surveys in the United States, England, and Wales showed that takers of oral contraceptive and menopausal hormones are at increased risk of suicide and mental illness.[111] There may be many reasons for this increased risk, such as the following:

- Natural or pharmaceutical changes in hormonal levels can lead to mood swings.
- Women seeking HRT may have health problems to begin with, although women in lower socioeconomic groups have more mental illness and are less likely to take HRT.
- HRT users may have higher expectations and consequently more disappointments and frustration.
- Hormone medications alter vitamin and mineral status, which can affect behavior.
- Interactions between hormones and other drugs may make symptoms worse. These other drugs include benzodiazepines (sedatives) or even moderate amounts of alcohol and coffee.

Surgery

Women should be advised to stop taking HRT four to six weeks before major surgery; relatively few women get this advice, however, and it is not possible in an emergency.

After examining twenty-nine menopausal women experiencing troublesome uterine bleeding while taking hormones, one expert suggests that if the bleeding is not controlled by changing the HRT regime, an effective alternative is to surgically remove the uterus so that the woman can continue HRT.[112] Surely a better option than surgery is to come off the hormones.

Surveys

A number of medical articles on HRT are based on surveys of women, and statistics are gathered from medical centers, government agencies, sales figures, and sometimes questionnaires or interviews. (These statistics are known as epidemiological evidence.) It is very difficult to interpret this type of information, which is why some experts say that this evidence should be considered interesting and worthy of follow-up but does not stand alone.

Women who respond to questionnaires, attend menopause clinics, or go to seminars tend to belong to higher socioeconomic groups than other women. Therefore, the information obtained is probably nonrepresentative. These women are more likely to take HRT, have healthier diets and lifestyles, more medical screenings, and less disease risk. Aside from higher socioeconomic standing, HRT users tend to be different from nonusers in a number of other ways; all these factors need to be considered.

Another underexamined issue is that women who take HRT tend to be former oral contraceptive users. From firsthand reports, women with breast cancer are asked if they have taken hormones. They may have taken oral contraceptives, but this may not be reported or was considered to be "too long ago to be relevant." The history of hormones indicates that adverse effects, notably cancer, can occur decades (even a generation) after hormone use, yet another reason why I suggest that the link between reproductive hormone therapies and cancer is underestimated.

Also, many women, particularly in the top socioeconomic group, take supplements and herbs but are reluctant to discuss them with their physicians. Because supplements and herbs can markedly reduce menopausal symptoms and improve bone mineral density, it is possible that these other compounds may be influencing the survey outcomes.

Surveys may not take into account the varying dosages and different types of hormones prescribed; many women also try a number of different regimes. In addition, looking at older studies may not be relevant to current prescribing practices.

Symptoms and Relationship to Estrogen Levels

Although HRT usually reduces symptoms such as flushing, night sweats, and vaginal dryness, some women have these symptoms even though their estrogen levels are relatively high. One study showed that external patches gave the same symptom relief as the stronger implants.[113]

When HRT does not help, sometimes the physician's mind-set is such that other causes of these symptoms (for example, fevers and infections cause sweating, and you can get vaginal dermatitis) are overlooked.

Thrombophilia (Blood Clots)

The risk of thrombophilia, or blood clots, is reportedly greater for women on oral contraceptives than for women not on them. With HRT, the magnitude and level of risk is uncertain.[114] At least three studies show that HRT estrogens are associated with an increased risk of blood clots, one of which was detailed in this chapter under the heading "Heart Disease, Hormones, and Women."

There are no data on the safety of estrogen patches for women who already have thrombosis. A further complication is that calcium supplementation by itself is associated with a risk of blood clots.[115] In other words, the combination of estrogen and calcium may further increase the risk of clots, yet it is commonly promoted.

A particular type of brain thrombosis is a rare but dangerous complication of HRT.[116]

Tinnitus and Deafness

Isolated cases of tinnitus (ringing in the ears) and deafness have been linked to HRT. The researchers in one case suggested that these cases may be due to estrogens disturbing mineral balance or alterations in neurotransmitters (nerve chemicals).[117]

Urinary Tract Infections

A study of 276 women concluded that estrogen use was associated with an increased risk of urinary tract infections in older women who still had a uterus, but not in women who had undergone hysterectomies.[118]

Uterus Problems

HRT users have six times more fibroids than nonusers, and hysterectomies are more common. Other uterine problems are discussed in the "Endometrial Disorders" section on page 40.

Vitamins, Minerals, and Other Nutrients

The beneficial effects of HRT on LDL cholesterol were reduced when estradiol valerate was combined with vitamin D (cholecalciferol).[119] Many women on HRT are told to take vitamin D and calcium supplementation, but this combination might cause more clots and an unhealthy lipid status.

A group of women treated with Premarin and progestin (medroxy-progesterone) were found to excrete higher than normal levels of zinc and magnesium.[120] Because zinc and magnesium are important for bone health, this detrimental interaction requires further investigation.

A U.K. medical specialist writes that HRT estrogens may cause surges in blood fats and increased copper levels, with lower serum zinc, folic acid, and essential fatty acid deficiency. She also states that estrogens are more powerful when combined with saturated fats.[121] Estrogen also reduces the body's vitamin C levels.

Well-Being

A study of Chinese women found general well-being was not affected by the absence of HRT, and the researchers issued a caution against universal HRT for postmenopausal women if quality of life is valued as a result.[122]

Youthfulness Claims

My favorite story is of a survey carried out in the United States. At a fitness center, used by a number of middle-aged women, researchers posted a notice for women to attend brief interviews concerning their experience of taking or avoiding hormone replacement therapy. Prior to the interviews the researchers privately jotted down their guesses of the women's ages. Subsequently, those not using HRT were three times more often judged to be younger than the guessed age. Curiously, when interviewed, the hormone users imagined that they looked young for their ages.

Some experiments show that compared with estrogen or progestin, testosterone and other anabolic steroids are more effective at strengthening the skin and other supporting structures of postmenopausal women; the effects taper off after three months, however, which means there is no justification for using any hormone drug to enhance your appearance, especially if it causes a lot of facial hair!

In twenty years, I've recommended HRT to very few of my patients. One memorable case was a seventy-year-old vegetarian woman (who looked about a hundred years old) whose main complaint was a dry vagina. She had recently remarried, to a much younger man, and was finding it painful to have sex. When I examined her, it was obvious that her vaginal tissue had been painful and itchy for many years. Her body was evidently not producing enough estrogen to keep her skin and other body tissues healthy, and this condition was exacerbated by a chronic and extremely low-fat diet. She was reluctant to use any form of pharmaceutical but tried an internal and external herbal and essential fatty acid program (fish oil, evening primrose oil, and vitamin E) without success. An estriol cream prescribed by a doctor markedly improved her vaginal tissue.

Even estriol (Ovestin), probably the gentlest of the estrogens, has a list of over fifty contraindications, cautions, warnings, and side effects. The majority of these problems may be somewhat theoretical and based on what actually occurs with more potent pharmaceuticals. These potential problems, however, serve as a reminder that all natural and pharmaceutical hormones are very potent chemicals, that they interact with one another and work on a feedback mechanism, and that they will compromise health if they are administered inappropriately.

If you have osteoporosis, seek medical advice. You can either follow a natural therapies program that will require taking supplements plus exercise and lifestyle improvements, and in one or two years you can have a bone scan to evaluate its effectiveness. Or, you can take a pharmaceutical and be guided by your physician.

HRT does not make you healthy. What makes you healthy is a sound diet, lifestyle, environment, education, effective coping skills, financial independence, and a certain amount of genetic luck. When a pill is invented that will relieve menopausal symptoms and prevent degenerative aging conditions such as osteoporosis and heart disease without adverse effects, I will take it myself and recommend it to other women. Meanwhile, follow the recommendations in this book to gain your best natural health.

CHAPTER THREE

Plants with Beneficial
Estrogenic Activity

A number of plant hormones, or phytoestrogens (*phyto* means "plant"), have the capacity to mimic the actions of the body. These compounds lower the body's estrogens when the levels are high and also provide some estrogenic activity when the levels are low, as is the case in menopausal women. This chapter provides information about how to use these plants to help relieve menopausal symptoms and prevent premature degenerative diseases and aging.

Every plant contains estrogen-like hormones and other types of hormones; they are required for the growth, sexual development, and survival of the plant itself.

In the very early stages of growth, the hormonal content of plants is high. It tapers off during growth and resurges when the plant is mature and producing seeds. The hormonal content is also affected by factors such as soil type, climate, and pest attacks. Because plants are not standard, one crop can be stronger than another.

One theory about how phytoestrogens were discovered is that farmers first noticed that certain plants caused an increase in milk production or fertility changes in animals. Scientists then applied this information to humans. The first scientific paper on phytoestrogens was published in 1927; since then, over ninety phytoestrogens have been identified in more than 300 plants. Thousands of papers have now been published on this topic.

By the 1940s, researchers in Australia and New Zealand observed that when sheep grazed on clover they became infertile. Scientists subsequently discovered that clover contains compounds called isoflavones that were similar to human estrogens, and that these compounds were the cause of the infertility in grazing animals.

These phytoestrogens are not the same as human estrogens, they are weaker, and, of course, humans do not eat pounds of raw clover on a daily basis. Phytoestrogens in human dietary quantities are nothing like contraceptive hormones.

PHYTOESTROGENS IN GENERAL

The most important phytoestrogens for menopausal women are

1. Isoflavones, notably genistein, daidzein, formononetin, and biochanin-A
2. Lignans

You will get a good supply of phytoestrogens if you eat the following foods regularly in normal dietary quantities:

- Soybeans and most soy products
- Sprouts, such as alfalfa
- Flaxseeds (linseed)
- Legumes (lentils, chickpeas, beans, peas)
- Whole grains
- Seeds, especially pumpkin, sunflower, and sesame
- Vegetables and fruits

Other useful foods and herbs are covered in this chapter as well as in chapters 4 and 5.

Generally, the protein part of soybeans and other legumes, and the fiber portion of grains and most seeds, are the best sources of phytoestrogens. If you eat white flour or white rice, for example, you won't be getting phyto-estrogens.

Isoflavones

Most phytoestrogenic plants contain variable quantities of the four main isoflavones: genistein, daidzein, biochanin-A, and formononetin. Glycetein is now emerging as another therapeutic isoflavonic phytoestrogen; this compound is found in soy. In the body, biochanin-A and formononetin can be converted to genistein and daidzein, respectively, and daidzein can be converted to equol.

Some of these valuable conversions do not take place if your intestinal bacteria are not in balance, if you have an inflammatory intestinal disorder, or if your diet is high in animal fats. Furthermore, antibiotics completely suppress these intestinal conversions.

How Isoflavones Balance Estrogens   Any type of estrogen needs to bind to receptors in your body to be used. Some of the isoflavones bind to hormone receptors even though they are much weaker than the body's estrogens. Thus, to a certain extent, isoflavones have the capacity to crowd out some of your body's stronger estrogens. A young woman who produces plenty of estradiol will get a beneficial antiestrogenic effect from plant estrogens, because they do not have the same capacity to stimulate new cells. In this way isoflavones may reduce the risk of cancer. When menstruating women were given 400 milliliters daily of soy milk containing 109 milligrams isoflavones, estradiol levels were reduced 27 percent and estrone was reduced 23 percent, whereas those who didn't get the soy milk had only slight increases.[1] On the other hand, when you are menopausal and your estrogen levels are very low, the phytoestrogens are more readily picked up by receptors and a degree of estrogen activity occurs.

The following is a very brief overview of the therapeutic benefits of isoflavones; there are well over 2,000 scientific papers published on isoflavones.

- Menopausal symptoms, compared with placebo and "tincture of time" are reduced. One controlled study found that 45 grams of soy flour per day could reduce the occurrence of flushes by 40 percent over twelve weeks.[2] My clinical experience over twenty years is that a combination of diet, herbs, and exercise gives a much greater improvement in menopause symptoms and well-being than one food or supplement.
- The quality of vaginal tissue is improved.[3]
- There is a potential to increase bone mineral density. Daily intake of 90 grams (a little over 3 ounces) of soy protein, which contains isoflavones, plus modest calcium supplementation produced a significant increase in bone mineral density after six months.[4] Another study showed that a soy-enriched diet containing 52 milligrams of isoflavones also improved bone mineral density, as did four slices of soy and linseed bread per day. Some studies indicate that Japanese women and vegetarian women sustain fewer fractures because of their isoflavone-rich diet, although various lifestyle factors may also be involved.
- A number of studies have shown that ipriflavone, a synthetic flavonoid, has the capacity to improve bone mineral density. Ipriflavone is covered in more detail in chapter 6.
- If you have osteoporosis and have been consuming a phytoestrogen-rich diet, my clinical studies based on bone mineral density scans show that adding more phytoestrogen will not help your bones. Also, animal studies show that the body adapts to phytoestrogens, so after a time the therapeutic effect probably lessens.
- Isoflavones can lower LDL cholesterol in those with high levels, the quantity used in one trial being only 38 milligrams of isoflavones (in 25 grams of soy protein).[5] The protein and other compounds in soy may be more valuable than isoflavones for lowering LDL cholesterol.
- Elasticity of arteries may be improved by consuming 40 to 80 milligrams isoflavones per day,[6] which is especially relevant to postmenopausal women because increasing age means loss of elasticity in the blood vessel walls.

- Isoflavones have antioxidant activity, including reduced DNA oxidation, which partly accounts for their role as natural cancer-protective compounds.[7] Isoflavones have various anticancer activities and may also reduce oxidation of the bad cholesterol.
- Brain circulation may be improved.[8]
- Many scientific papers support the notion that a diet rich in soy and isoflavones appears to reduce the incidence of cancer, particularly breast, prostate, and colon cancers.[9]
- The evidence for breast cancer is supported by many dietary surveys and at least three studies of urinary excretion of phytoestrogens confirming a substantial reduction in breast cancer risk in women with a high phytoestrogen intake.[10] One author has referred to studies on genistein and other soy isoflavones; and there were more than 132 listed research papers, many in respect to cancer prevention.[11] All we need now are large-scale trials on humans.
- Japanese people have the longest life span of people from any nation. According to the World Health Organization, they also appear to have the best quality of life at seventy years of age. Traditionally, Japanese have been the largest consumers of soy and have intakes of isoflavones varying between 20 and 300 milligrams daily. The lower incidence of reproductive cancers in Japan may be related to long-term use of isoflavone-rich foods as well as other dietary and lifestyle factors, but it is known that when Japanese adopt an American diet they also take on the U. S. rates of cancer.

Warnings About Isoflavones   Despite some criticism of isoflavones and soy foods related to their hormonal effects—especially in infants—there is no substantial evidence to support harm from normal dietary quantities of isoflavone-rich foods or soy formulas fed to infants, which has been practiced since the 1970s. (Breast milk, however, is best for babies.)

Studies with most animals and studies with all birds are unlikely to be relevant because isoflavones are not a normal part of those diets and those creatures metabolize estrogens differently than humans. Be aware that compared with human dietary intakes, animals in laboratory studies or grazing have consumed enormous quantities of isoflavones.

There are some warnings, however, about isoflavones.

- Isoflavonic foods in excess quantities may reduce thyroid activity. People on thyroxine medication should not eat isoflavone-rich foods within three hours of taking medication. Isoflavone-rich foods include soybeans and soy products, all sprouts, and isoflavone products. There is no hard evidence that the quantities of isoflavones in whole grains and herbs interfere with thyroid metabolism, but that is entirely possible. If you are on thyroid medication, discuss diet and supplements with your physician.
- Women with breast cancer who are taking Tamoxifen should not have a diet rich in phytoestrogens or take isoflavone supplements unless advised by their physician because it is uncertain how these two interact. They are both able to occupy estrogen receptor sites in the body.
- A number of scientists have expressed concern about the role of isoflavones in health and the following is the consensus of the North American Menopause Society.

> Although the observed health effects in humans cannot be clearly attributed to isoflavones alone, it is clear that foods or supplements that contain isoflavones have some physiologic effects. Clinicians may wish to recommend that menopausal women consume whole foods that contain isoflavones, especially for the cardiovascular benefits of these foods; however, a level of caution needs to be observed in making these recommendations. Additional clinical trials are needed before specific recommendations can be made regarding increased consumption of foods or supplements that contain high amounts of isoflavones.[12]

The same cautions could be given for every food, herb, and drink, given that they all contain numerous compounds that have biological effects in humans. There will never be sufficient studies. Hundreds of studies have been done on single hormone compounds, and the experts are still asking for more evidence. It is unfeasible to assess the 500 or so compounds in every plant to see how they affect the body and how they interact with the many thousands of compounds we take in every day. The only sensible option for the majority of people is to eat a wide variety of foods in as natural a state as possible. The overwhelming bulk of evidence shows that isoflavone-rich foods are health-enhancing. The following foods and herbs are rich sources of isoflavones:

- Soybeans
- All sprouts
- Clovers
- Alfalfa
- Whole grains
- Hops
- Sage
- Black cohosh
- Parsley and probably most herbs in this family (Apiaceae), such as caraway, chervil, coriander, cumin, dill, lovage, and possibly carrots and parsnips
- Licorice
- Most legumes, including chickpeas, mung beans, and lentils

A few researchers have suggested that a number of other flavonoid compounds have weak estrogenic effects.[13] These compounds are found in fresh fruits, vegetables, nuts, seeds, herbs, and dried fruit.

The quantities of isoflavones needed for therapeutic purposes are indicated later in this chapter.

Lignans

Lignans are found in the fibrous outer portion of plants. Although there are many different types of lignans, this section will only cover those known to have phytoestrogenic activity in humans.

These compounds are excreted in large quantities in the urine, which means that they need to be consumed regularly for a therapeutic effect. Like isoflavones, if the phytoestrogenic lignans are not used immediately, they are apparently rapidly excreted so that there is no harmful build up. Antibiotics and a high-fat diet prevent the body's beneficial conversion of these lignans.

The phytoestrogenic lignans are modified by intestinal bacteria to form compounds such as enterolactone and enterodiol, which are then absorbed into the body. They have estrogen-balancing effects similar to isoflavones as well as anticancer and antioxidant activity.[14]

Dietary lignans have been linked to a lowered incidence of breast cancer, as illustrated in table 3.1.

Lignans have been shown to have antiviral, antitumor, anti-inflammatory, and antiallergy properties and may have a protective effect on the heart and circulatory systems.[15]

Foods Sources of Phytoestrogenic Lignans Ground flaxseed (meal) is by far the best source of lignans. Smaller quantities are found in flaxseed oil, pumpkin seeds, cranberry, sunflower seeds, sesame seeds, mung bean sprouts, broccoli, garlic, carrots, grain fiber, buckwheat, soy fiber, legumes, dried seaweed, and most seeds and berries. A number of vegetables and fruits contain tiny quantities of these lignans.

TABLE 3.1 **Enterolactone Content of Urine**

Dietary group	Parts per million/liter
Macrobiotic	17,680
Lactovegetarians	4,170
Meat-eaters	2,050
Postmenopausal breast cancer patients	1,040

Adapted from: Adlercreutz, H., et al. "Determination of Urinary Lignans and Phytoestrogen Metabolites, Potential Antiestrogens and Anticarcinogens, in Urine of Women on Various Habitual Diets," *Journal of Steroid Biochemistry* 25 (1986): 791.

Note: Breast cancer patients also have lower levels of equol (an isoflavone metabolite) and higher levels of human estrogens.

Sesame seed contains a lignan (sesamin) that protects vitamin E in the body and reduces the oxidation of fats in the body.[16]

Coumestrol

Coumestrol is the collective name for the over twenty coumestans that have been identified to date. According to laboratory tests, they are the strongest phytoestrogens. In animals, coumestrol reduces FSH and LH, the two hormones that are high in menopausal and postmenopausal women. Coumestrol competes for binding to the estrogen receptor, so it may also balance hormones similar to isoflavones. A coumestrol derivative also improved the bones of animals.[17]

The best sources of coumestrol are soy and alfalfa sprouts and to a lesser extent legumes, including green beans, split peas, and red beans.

Coumarins, which are similar to coumestrol, have anticlotting (anticoagulant) activity, but there is no evidence that foods rich in coumestrol have this ability in any measurable extent in the human body. If you are on anticoagulant drugs, however, avoid sprouts and discuss your diet and supplements with your physician.

Other Plant Hormones

Zearalenone (a resorcylic acid lactone) is a fungal estrogen known to bind to estrogen sites. This compound appears to be effective in treating menopausal symptoms.[18]

These estrogens occur naturally in some foods and there is no evidence that they adversely affect humans, although it is advisable to avoid fungally infected foods. American and Australian marketable corn—as well as wheat, barley, sorghum, rice, and other grains—contain these estrogens, and high concentrations occur when grains are stored in warm, humid conditions.

Gibberellic acid is a common plant hormone. It is not known whether the tiny quantities in foods have any effects in humans, although in rat studies gibberellic acid produced reproductive and growth effects and also reduced tumor growth. It is probably nonactive in the quantities that humans would consume.

Phytosterols (Plant Steroids)

Phytosterols are hormone-like substances present in all plants. There are about sixty different types of phytosterols. The most common, and likely to be beneficial to humans, are beta-sitosterol, stigmasterol, and camposterol. Studies in animals show that when used as isolated compounds, these phytosterols have estrogenic effects.[19]

Phytosterols help lower blood cholesterol by competing with cholesterol for absorption. They are a common component of plant foods consumed in relatively large quantities by vegetarians, who are at lower risk for colon and reproductive cancers.[20]

Food Sources of Phytosterols

- Plant oils, especially corn, sesame, safflower, and wheat germ (the majority of plant oils contain from 100 to 500 milligrams sterol per 100 grams)
- Rice bran and whole grains
- Nuts and seeds, including chestnuts and sesame, safflower, sunflower, and pumpkin seeds
- Legumes contain from 23 to 220 milligrams per 100 grams
- Vegetables contain between 1 and 200 milligrams sterol per 100 grams. Most of the high values for vegetables are for seedlings (vegelets), and ways of growing and using these as food are given in chapter 4.

Herbal Sources of Phytosterols   Traditional hormone herbs contain phytosterols, and it is probable that when the body's estrogens are low these plant hormones have some therapeutic effects. Some herbs in this category include:

- Calendula
- Chaparral
- Dandelion
- Dong quai
- Ginseng
- Psyllium
- St. John's wort
- Saw palmetto
- Valerian

See chapter 5 for more information on specific phytoestrogenic and menopausal herbs.

Gamma oryzanol is a particular category of phytosterol that has been used as a medicine in Japan since 1962. It is effective for treating menopause symptoms, including hot flashes, by reducing LH and promoting the release of endorphins in the brain; that is, it increases well-being hormones. It produces a number of effects on pituitary and hypothalamus control hormones but does not appear to alter the level of hormones they control. It also reduces LDL and triglyceride levels. In addition, gamma oryzanol has healing and soothing effects on the digestive system and is an antioxidant.[21] Animal studies show that gamma oryzanol decreases fatty deposits in the arteries by as much as 67 percent.[22]

Contrary to some promotional material, there is no evidence that gamma oryzanol is a body-building substance, but it is an underutilized compound in Western countries given its many therapeutic advantages.

The most abundant food sources of gamma oryzanol are rice bran oil and other grain oils such as corn oil and barley oil. It is also present in many foods, such as whole rice, oats, berries, citrus fruits, tomatoes, olives, and vegetables. Rice bran is quite high in chemical residues, so try to buy organic rice bran products. If you are constipated, add 10 to 20 grams of rice bran to your breakfast cereal and get all the other benefits!

Do Plants Contain Human Hormones?

Yes, plants do contain human hormones, according to early studies and a phytochemical dictionary.[23] With the exception of common green beans which are said to contain minute amounts of estradiol, however, the other plants—for example, pomegranate seeds and pussy willow flowers—are not edible.

SUPER PHYTOESTROGENIC FOODS

The Benefits of Soy

Soybeans contain over 500 constituents, and at least a dozen books have been written solely on this food. There are more than 7,000 published scientific reports for soy and its components, and the overwhelming bulk of them support soy as a health-enhancing food.

It is best to consume whole foods rather than concentrated isoflavones, because a whole plant contains many therapeutic compounds such as lignans, phytosterols, essential fatty acids, saponins, and nutrients. Evidence shows that people who have eaten soybeans and soy products for long periods of time enjoy better-than-average health. Table 3.2 lists soy products currently available.

Reduces Menopausal Flushing   A 45 percent reduction in flushes was achieved with a daily intake of 60 grams of isolated soy protein; a similar reduction in night sweats was noted.[24] Most studies had a duration of up to twelve weeks and used between 45 to 60 grams of a soy product relatively high in isoflavones. My experience is that severe symptoms often need a combination of diet, herbs, and exercise, and some women may need to take an additional concentrated supplement to get relief.

Improves Vaginal Tissue   Soy has been shown to improve the texture of vaginal lining in some women.[25]

Lowers Breast Cancer Risk   A study in China found that women with breast cancer had lower levels of phytoestrogens in their urine compared with women who did not have cancer.[26] Soy is the main source of isoflavonoids in Asian countries.

General Cancer Prevention   The death rate from prostate, colon, and possibly other cancers might be reduced with increased consumption of soybean products. Laboratory and animal experiments show that soy contains a number of cancer-preventing compounds including phytates, flavonoids, carotenoids, trypsin inhibitors, saponins, and genistein.[27] This finding supports a number of large dietary surveys relating to cancer prevention.

Cholesterol- and Triglyceride-Lowering Properties   After studying thirty-seven reports, a group of researchers concluded that eating soy protein markedly decreased total cholesterol, LDL cholesterol, and triglycerides.[28] Soy isoflavones also have the capacity to improve arterial elasticity. Improving circulation in this way is likely to bring about far reaching benefits to the body.

TABLE 3.2 **Types of Soy Products Available**

Soy Product	Characteristics
Dried soybeans	*Basic cooking method:*
	Place 2 cups soybeans with 8 cups water in a large saucepan.
	Bring to boil, then turn off heat.
	Allow to cool, then drain water.
	Add another 8 cups water.
	Bring to boil and simmer until tender, usually more than two hours (a pressure cooker or microwave speeds the cooking time).
	They need flavoring or can be added to soups and casseroles.
	Another option is to roast the cooked beans in the oven until they are dry and crunchy, then flavor with herbs and a low-sodium soy sauce.
Fresh soybeans	Cook like green peas. Soak in boiling water for about five minutes to extract the beans from the pods. You'll be surprised how tasty they are.
Soy milk and yogurt	Use as dairy substitutes.
Soy flour	Too heavy to be used by itself in most recipes but generally can be substituted for about one-quarter of wheat flour. It must be cooked.
Soy sprouts	Also surprisingly tasty but need a little cooking, either in stir-fries or steamed, or cooled and added to salads.
Dried tofu (bean curd)	Needs to be softened in water before cooking.

(continued overleaf)

TABLE 3.2 (*continued*)

Soy Product	Characteristics
Firm tofu	Usually sold packaged in a little liquid and requires refrigeration. Has the texture of soft rubber and should be flavored with other foods or herbs and spices. It is often sliced and marinated before adding to stir-fries. Tofu takes on the taste of whatever it is cooked with. Can be mashed into burgers.
Silken tofu	The most suitable tofu for blending and use in mayonnaise and desserts.
Tempeh	Taste and texture are similar to cold pork sausage. Use grated over salads or thinly sliced into stir-fries. It also requires flavoring.
Textured vegetable protein (TVP)	Soak in water and then use like ground meat.
Soy flakes	Suitable to add to porridge, in cookies, or as a thickening agent in casseroles.
Soy grits	May be cooked with rice or added to soups.
Miso	A salty, dark-colored paste derived from fermenting soy. Often used for flavoring soups; it can also be used as a spread on bread (resembles the famous Australian Vegemite, a sandwich spread unappreciated in other countries). Miso is used fairly sparingly, about a teaspoon per serving. You won't get any estrogenic effect from this quantity, but it is a healthy condiment.
Soy sauces	Various types, including salt-reduced tamari, are available.

TABLE 3.2 (*continued*)	
Soy Product	*Characteristics*
Soy cheese	Texture is somewhat rubbery and not as tasty as dairy cheese, but I use an herb-flavored variety grated into salads. It's also excellent grilled on toast and tomato, especially if you spread it with miso first.
Other soy products	You can buy or make tofu ice cream and desserts. Soy pasta, noodles, schnitzels, hot dogs, cookies, coffee, chips, roasted soy nuts, and various snack forms of soy are also available commercially.

Benefits to the Digestive System   Although many people find soy difficult to digest, especially if it is not properly cooked, fermented, or processed, the carbohydrates in it tend to support an increase in healthy bacteria in the bowel. Soybean fiber prevents constipation, and when added to cereals it gives a better control of blood glucose.[29]

Nutritional Benefits   Soy is a good source of essential amino acids and fatty acids. It is rich in minerals and vitamins, with the exception of vitamin B_{12}. Tempeh, however, a fermented soy product, can contain this vitamin, but it depends on how the tempeh is manufactured. Soybeans are very inexpensive relative to their nutritional and health advantages, although some processed products, such as soy cheese, are more expensive than dairy cheese.

Isolated components, such as isoflavones in soy, may not be as effective as the food itself because the whole food contains a number of therapeutic compounds.

Cautions

- Soy is a fairly common allergen and must be avoided if you are sensitive to it.

83

- People on cancer therapy should discuss their diet with a practitioner. A high soy diet might interfere with some types of hormonal cancer drugs, such as Tamoxifen.
- Trypsin inhibitors in uncooked soybeans prevent protein uptake, but they are markedly reduced when soy is properly cooked. These compounds, however, have anticancer activity.
- Some of the carbohydrates in soy cause intestinal gas if not adequately cooked. Raw soybeans need to be soaked and cooked until soft. These same carbohydrates, however, have the capacity to increase beneficial bacteria in the intestines.
- A number of people find soy hard to digest, so I recommend small quantities to start. In addition, always use herbs for flavoring and to help with digestion.
- Phytic acid (in soy, grains, legumes, and other foods) is said to reduce mineral absorption. If you are on a healthy diet, however, your mineral intake should be more than adequate, and laboratory studies show that phytic acid has cancer-preventing properties.
- The preponderance of evidence supports that soy is cancer preventive or cancer protective, but no large-scale controlled study has been done.
- Soy is not appropriate for household pets and most animals, just as a diet solely of raw meat is not appropriate for humans.
- See the additional cautions listed under isoflavones on page 74.

Although soy infant formulas have been criticized and some may have been nutritionally inadequate in the past, medical researchers state that they are not aware of "any epidemiological or clinical evidence to support the contention that the current level of exposure of human infants to isoflavones from natural diets or soy formulas has adverse effects. Indeed, it is possible that a moderate level of exposure is beneficial."[30]

All plants contain around 500 different compounds, some of which are classified as naturally occurring toxins. In general, if you eat a varied diet, you should get a good range of beneficial compounds and avoid a harmful buildup of particular toxins. The numerous manufactured chemicals in our food and environment and the increasing number of hormonal drugs are a far greater concern.

Some Soy Recipes

SOY MENOPAUSE PORRIDGE
Serves 1

4 tablespoons soy flakes
2 tablespoons rye flakes or substitute
1 tablespoon sunflower seeds or 8 almonds
1 tablespoon dried raisins
1 tablespoon whey powder
1 cup water

Simmer for about five minutes, turn off the heat, and let stand for five minutes.

Serve with concentrated juice and soy yogurt.

TOFU OR TEMPEH
Serves 4 as a meat extender or substitute

¼ pound (2 cups) tofu or tempeh cut into cubes about ½-inch square
1 tablespoon corn oil (or other oil)
1 tablespoon low-sodium tamari (or other soy sauce)
1 teaspoon lemon juice or vinegar (see herbal vinegar recipe on page 96)
1 tablespoon curry powder or a selection of your favorite dried herbs
1 clove garlic, crushed (optional)

Place all ingredients in a baking dish and stir together. Place in the oven and roast for about ten minutes at 350°F (180°C). The tofu can be added hot to stir-fries or casseroles, or cold to salads.

EASY SOY COOKIES (MINI MUFFINS)
Makes 12

1 cup soy flour
½ cup self-rising whole meal flour
½ cup sesame seeds

½ cup sultanas or raisins
½ cup pumpkin seeds or almonds, chopped
I cup soy milk
I cup blueberries or I green apple, peeled and grated

Combine all the dry ingredients. Add the soy milk and mix thoroughly. Spoon the mixture into a well-greased cookie tray. Place the blueberries or grated apple on top.

Bake for twenty minutes at 350°F (180°C), then turn the oven to 280°F (120°C) and bake for another ten minutes.

Tofu Berry Mousse
Serves 4

10 ounces silken (soft) tofu
2 cups fresh or frozen berries
2 tablespoons rice syrup or concentrated apple juice
2 tablespoons cashews or almonds, ground

Blend the ingredients together until smooth. Pour into four small bowls or serving glasses. Chill before serving.

Optional: Sprinkle top with sesame seeds and a whole berry.

Most manufacturers of soy products supply recipes. If you find them bland, be adventurous and try adding more flavorings.

Flaxseed, Linseed (*Linum usitatissimum*)

The lignans in flaxseed are important for relieving menopausal symptoms, and they are scientifically supported as cancer-preventing compounds. Flaxseed lignans are known to beneficially modify estrogens and testosterone in the body, and dietary intake is linked to a lower incidence of breast, prostate, and uterine cancers.

A diet that contains one-fourth the caloric intake as soybeans and flaxseed will reduce hot flashes and vaginal dryness and will promote beneficial changes in hormone biochemistry, such as increased sex hormone binding globulin levels.[31] It may be difficult to eat this quantity for more than a few weeks, although a wider variety of phytoestrogen-rich foods could easily be consumed.

Flaxseed compounds have antioxidant activity, lower LDL cholesterol, and may prevent atherosclerosis.[32] A six-week scientifically controlled study showed that 1.3 ounces of flaxseed daily for six weeks lowered LDL cholesterol by 15 percent in postmenopausal women.[33]

Flaxseed is high in soluble fiber and is a good source of beneficial omega-3 fatty acids, both of which may contribute to the known beneficial effects on the body's fats. The type of lignans found in flaxseed have the capacity to prevent blood clumping (antiplatelet), relax blood vessels, and reduce blood pressure.[34]

Animal studies confirm the colon cancer protective effect of flaxseed.[35] In rats, 5 percent flaxseed added to the diet reduces both the initiation and growth of breast cancer due to the alpha-linolenic acid (oil) content and a lignan.[36] Naturopaths have long recommended flaxseed for constipation and colon health. One study showed that bowel movements per week increased by 30 percent from a daily consumption of 50 grams.[37] I have also found it helpful in treating some skin problems, such as psoriasis.

Other studies have shown that flaxseed may be helpful in treating lupus and the kidney problems associated with that disease as well as rheumatoid arthritis, mainly because of the types of oils it contains, notably alpha-linolenic acid.[38]

Recommended Quantity   I generally recommend about 10 to 20 grams of ground flaxseed daily, along with other lignan-rich foods regularly. If you don't have menopause symptoms and are not constipated, you can use less if it is not palatable to you.

How to Use Flaxseed   I recommend it in the form of ground seed (meal); commercial bread with whole seeds, however, apparently also releases the phytoestrogenic lignans in the body.

Add the seeds, or meal, to cereals, porridges, cookies, muffins, and burgers.

Avoid adding flaxseed in any form to soups or casseroles because it has a gluelike consistency and spoils the appearance and texture of the meal.

Flaxseed oil should be purchased in small quantities and kept in dark bottles in the refrigerator. If it goes rancid or is heated, the chemistry of the oil changes and it is no longer beneficial.

FLAXSEED AND SOY BURGERS
Makes 12 small burgers (for six people as a meat substitute)

This recipe is a basic burger or loaf mix. You can make up your own version, using soy flakes, nuts and seeds, cooked rice, and lentils as well as various vegetables.

1 onion, finely chopped
1 sweet potato, peeled and diced
½ cup soy milk
2 cups flaxseed meal
2 cups rye flakes (or cooked whole-grain rice)
½ cup walnut pieces
2 to 3 tablespoons dried fresh herbs (chives, parsley, basil, mint, oregano),
    or 1 to 2 teaspoons curry powder or mixed dried herbs and garlic
1 tablespoon low-sodium tamari
1 egg, beaten

Cook the onion and peeled diced sweet potato in a large saucepan with 1 cup water. (If you use the saucepan as a mixing bowl, it saves the washing.)

Mash the potato and onion mixture with the soy milk. Add the flaxseed meal, rye flakes, herbs, walnuts, and tamari. Mix thoroughly. Add the beaten egg to the mix. (To prevent the burgers from falling apart, let the mix stand for an hour or so in the refrigerator.)

Form into burgers, covering the outsides with millet meal or barley flakes. Place the burgers on a greased tray, painting the tops with a little olive oil. (When I'm in a hurry I make a loaf instead.)

Bake at 350°F for twenty-five minutes.

Serve hot with chopped, cooked tomatoes flavored with a little chili and some fresh chives, or use cold, broken into a salad.

FLAXSEED AND LIGNAN COOKIES
Makes about 30 cookies

5 heaping tablespoons tahini
5 heaping tablespoons honey
2 cups flaxseed meal
1 cup rye flakes
1 cup ground pumpkin seeds
1 cup dried black currants
½ cup sesame seeds or sunflower seeds
½ cup barley flakes
½ cup carob powder
½ cup dried coconut

Melt the tahini and honey in a large saucepan, but don't boil. Add all the other ingredients and mix together as best you can. Tip the mixture into a large greased baking dish. Flatten the mix firmly with your hands. If the mixture is hard to flatten, run your hands under cold water to prevent sticking and to moisten the mix.

Bake in a 300°F (140°C) oven for about twenty-five minutes.

When still slightly warm, cut into small squares. Store in the refrigerator.

You can substitute any type of whole grain flour, flakes, cornmeal, or whey powder and can add a little ginger and licorice powder. Ingredients can be varied to suit your taste.

If you find the cookies too rich, reduce the quantity of seeds. If you're constipated, substitute some rice bran. You can melt a large bar of carob and spread over the cookies while they are hot. These cookies are not low in calories, but they are useful as a healthy treat because they satisfy sweet cravings and are a good source of phytoestrogens and calcium.

Legumes

Phytoestrogenic legumes include peas, beans, lentils, and chickpeas. A number of legumes have been eaten by human beings for about 8,000 years. Unfortunately, as human beings became more "civilized," they began to eat less of them, and the legume became known as a "poor man's meat."

All legumes have some phytoestrogenic activity. Some of their general benefits are as follows:

- Legumes are high in fiber, thereby preventing constipation.
- Between 60 and 100 grams a day of legumes have the capacity to lower cholesterol by 7 to 26 percent in those with high cholesterol.[39]
- Glucose metabolism is often improved on diets rich in legumes.
- Legumes generally contain healthy oils, are a useful source of most of the B vitamins, and contain abundant potassium as well as relatively good quantities of iron, zinc, and magnesium.[40]

Cautions

- By themselves, legumes are not rich in all the essential amino acids (protein building blocks), but that can be overcome by having other foods rich in amino acids—such as meat, grains, nuts, corn, or dairy foods—in the same meal.
- Flour made from legumes must be cooked to reduce potentially harmful and indigestible components.
- To prevent digestive problems, all dried legumes are soaked and then cooked until soft. I always add digestive herbs and spices to them.

Recipes

LENTIL AND BARLEY CURRY
Serves 8

1 cup lentils
1 cup pearl barley
1 onion, chopped
4 cups vegetables, such as carrots, celery, or zucchini, chopped
    Curry powder or paste to taste (start with 1 tablespoon)
    Seasoning to taste

Check that there are no stones in the lentils. Wash the lentils.

Soak the lentils overnight in 3 cups water. Discard the water and wash again (not as important with lentils as with larger legumes). Add a further 3 cups of water to the lentils, bring to a boil, and simmer for thirty minutes.

Then add the barley, chopped onion, and curry and continue to cook for fifteen minutes while you prepare the vegetables. Add the vegetables and cook until they are soft.

For taste, add extra curry, herbs, or seasoning if required.

Serve with yogurt and finely chopped chives or parsley.

Variations: Put the cooked savory lentils and barley into a deep baking dish, add mashed potatoes to the top, sprinkle with soy or dairy cheese, and bake until the top is lightly browned. This variation is better flavored with herbs rather than curry.

Sometimes I mash cooked beans, add mashed tofu and eggs plus chopped nuts, vegetables, and herbs, and make into loaves or burgers.

Always use herbs and spices with any variation because legumes need flavoring and digestive support.

SPICY CHICKPEAS
Serves 4–6

2 cups chickpeas
1 tablespoon each of curry powder, vinegar, soy sauce, and oil
 (other herbs and seasonings may be substituted)

Soak chickpeas overnight in 6 cups water. Discard the water and wash the chickpeas.

Add a further 4 cups water and simmer for about three hours until the peas are soft but not mushy. The cooking time will be much faster if you use a pressure cooker or microwave.

Pour into a baking dish. Add curry powder, vinegar, soy sauce, oil, or your preferred herbs or flavorings. Mix together so that the flavorings are spread throughout the chickpeas.

Bake in the oven at 400°F (200°C) for about fifteen minutes.

Use hot in other dishes, cold in salads, or as a snack.

Whole Grains

Whole grains have many protective compounds, including isoflavonic phytoestrogens and lignans, fiber, antioxidants, and cancer-preventive compounds.[41]

ole grains contain a much higher level of vitamins and minerals—
nin E, selenium, zinc, and manganese—than refined products.
e fiber may reduce the uptake of some nutrients to a certain
extent, it is important to remember that the whole grain, together with its
fiber, contains considerably more nutrients to begin with and the fiber contains important anticancer components. The advantages clearly outweigh the
slight theoretical disadvantages.

In my clinic, I see many people who eat too much wheat, usually refined
products. Typically, they have a wheat cereal for breakfast, sandwiches for
lunch, and pasta for dinner, and they often have gastrointestinal or allergic
reactions.

I recommend consuming a variety of whole grains but not with every
meal, because a wide variety of foods should be eaten to give the widest benefits. At the most, you should have grains twice daily.

Some people are allergic or extremely sensitive to the gluten in wheat
and must avoid it; the same goes for rye, oats, barley, and triticale (a
wheat/rye cross). A number of wheat substitutes and grainlike foods do not
contain gluten, and most contain some phytoestrogens.

Wheat Substitutes

- Rye, oat, barley, and triticale all contain gluten. Rye, oat, and barley
  bran all help lower cholesterol and are useful as treatment for constipation. Rye bran has been shown in animal studies to reduce
  colon tumor development.[42]
- Rice and millet are gluten free and are relatively good sources of
  many essential nutrients, which explains why billions of people use
  these two grains as a staple food. Millet, unlike other grains, is not
  acid residue, which may account for its reputation as a suitable food
  for people with arthritis.
- Corn is a staple food in parts of Africa and South America. It com-
  plements beans in both agriculture and nutrition. If you combine
  corn with beans, the protein in that meal becomes more usable. For
  example, thicken bean dishes with cornmeal or have corn on the
  cob as an entrée followed by a bean casserole.

- Buckwheat (*Fagopyren repens*) is a gluten-free seed harvested from a shrub. It can be used in a similar way to most grains but does not take as long to cook. Buckwheat can be boring without added flavorsome foods, but it does contain phytoestrogenic lignans and is a rich source of rutin and other flavonoids. When you buy buckwheat, make sure that you buy the kernel (the inside part). The seeds have a brown, hard, outer coat that is very difficult to remove.

Grains and grainlike foods need cooking until soft. Most grains and many grain substitutes, such as legumes and various starchy foods, are available as flours, pasta, noodles, flakes, cookies, and even commercial breads.

Linseed, quinoa, and amaranth seeds can be ground into meal, which can then be used as a partial flour substitute. Remember that seeds contain valuable phytoestrogenic lignans and essential fatty acids, that is, the healthy fats.

Recipes The following few recipes demonstrate that there are numerous ways of getting a therapeutic intake of phytoestrogens.

In most recipes, you can substitute or partially substitute other grains or grainlike compounds. Use your imagination and culinary skills, but don't begin with too many variations.

BASIC PLAIN MILLET
Serves 4

I cup hulled millet (unhulled millet is virtually impossible to cook)
1¾ cups water

Bring the water to a boil and add the millet. Cover and simmer gently for twenty-five minutes.

It is better not to stir the millet, but check periodically, by putting a spoon down the inside of the saucepan, to see that it is not burning.

Turn off the heat and leave the lid on for about five minutes. Fluff with a fork before serving.

Millet is sweetish but somewhat bland. Serve with curried sweet potato, onion, and other vegetables.

Variations: Cooked millet can also be used in casseroles. Try combining it with cooked onion and spinach, and then add cheese, tomato, mushrooms, beaten egg, and a little grated nutmeg. Turn into a shallow baking dish, grate some soy cheese over the top, and broil for about ten minutes until light brown. Any grain or vegetable combination can be used in this way. To give more flavor, add herbs and seeds such as sesame or sunflower.

BARLEY PORRIDGE
Makes 1 large serving (to keep you going until lunchtime!)

½ cup whole grain barley
½ cup mixed dried fruit
1½ cups water

Bring the ingredients to a boil the night before, preferably in a heavy non-stick saucepan. Then turn off the heat and let stand overnight with the lid on. In the morning, heat and serve with milk, yogurt, or concentrated apple juice.

This method is a traditional way of making whole grain porridge. People used to heat it in a heavy pot and cover it with a blanket overnight.

Barley flakes don't require overnight soaking and are also quite good as a quick porridge.

I use barley flakes when kneading bread, as they make a crunchy crust. When I make soy burgers I often coat them with barley flakes. Pearl barley can be used as a rice substitute or cooked to make a tabouli substitute. Barley is one of the tastiest of the grains.

RYE AND BUCKWHEAT PIE CRUST
Serves 6

3 tablespoons tahini
3 tablespoons honey
1 cup rye flakes
1 cup buckwheat kernels
½ cup millet or soy flakes
½ cup blended walnuts or almonds
½ teaspoon vanilla essence

In a large pot, melt the honey and tahini (don't boil). Add all the other ingredients and mix thoroughly. Dip your hands in cold water and press the mix firmly into an oiled flan or pie dish.

Bake for ten minutes at 300°F. Remove from oven, cool, add cooked apples or lightly cooked berries.

I cook four apples in a little water until soft and add either 3 teaspoons gelatin powder or agar powder, or thicken with arrowroot flour. This way, the fruit on top of the crust will be firm when you serve it. If you use apples, lightly sprinkle cinnamon powder on top.

Bake for another twelve minutes at 300°F.

COLD BUCKWHEAT SALAD
Serves 4–6

½ cup onion, finely chopped
1 cup buckwheat kernels
2 cups water
½ avocado
1 tomato, finely chopped
1 cup mushrooms, finely chopped
½ cup dairy or soy yogurt
½ cup cashew nuts
½ cup fresh mixed herbs (parsley; chives; basil; rocket, a wonderful salad
    herb [like lettuce] with a nutty, tangy flavor) finely chopped
1 tablespoon low-sodium tamari or other flavoring
1 small-leafed lettuce

Bring the water to a boil, add the onion, and simmer for five minutes. Add the buckwheat and simmer for another five minutes.

When cool, gently combine all the ingredients except the lettuce. Place the mix in a serving bowl.

Wash and drain the lettuce leaves. Place the lettuce leaves on a separate plate.

People can serve themselves by putting about a tablespoon of the buckwheat salad mix onto a lettuce leaf and rolling it up to eat with their hands.

Seeds and Oils

Seeds and oils contain various categories of phytoestrogens and phytosterols, and a reasonable intake is about 1 tablespoon daily of either. A 1957 study showed that the vaginal tissue of postmenopausal women improved when they consumed 100 grams corn oil or olive oil daily for ten days.[43] This amount is far too much oil to consume daily, but a lesser amount consumed regularly should provide a healthy intake of essential fatty acids (oils) as well as the hormonal compounds.

The most recommended "menopause" seeds are flaxseed, sesame seeds, pumpkin seeds, and sunflower seeds. Olives also contain phytoestrogens and sterols. Oils are available from these products, but it is much more therapeutic to buy cold-pressed or virgin oil, to buy in small quantities, and not to heat the oil. I use some olive oil for cooking but avoid heating it excessively.

Cabbage   A German study showed that cabbage had more phytoestrogenic activity than red clover or peas.[44] It has been established in a number of surveys that eating normal dietary quantities of cabbage seems to protect people against various cancers.

All plants in the cabbage family contain glucosinolates, which release indole-3-carbinol, which in turn produces diindolymethane. This latter compound is said to promote good by-products of estrogen and prevent breast cancer in particular.[45]

A healthy way to include cabbage in the diet is the following:

Wash and finely shred cabbage leaves.

Pour a small quantity of herbal vinegar (about 2 teaspoons per person) over the cabbage.

Let stand about thirty to sixty minutes so that the vinegar makes the cabbage more easily digestible. Then add other salad ingredients such as grated carrot and savory tofu.

PHYTOESTROGENIC HERBAL VINEGAR

¾ pint apple cider, rice, or balsamic vinegar
1 large handful fresh phytoestrogenic herbs (such as sage, angelica, aniseed, caraway, dill, fennel, gotu kola, hops, licorice), chopped

2 teaspoons parsley or celery seeds, crushed
2 teaspoons dried ginger powder
2 teaspoons dried turmeric powder

The ginger and turmeric are for flavoring and digestion. Pour half the vinegar into a pint bottle or jar. Add the herbs and cover with the rest of the vinegar. Seal and store on its side for at least a few days before use. You can add all dried herbs if fresh ones are not available, but they swell considerably in the vinegar, so restrict the dried herbs to 12 teaspoons total.

The herbs and quantities can be varied according to your taste and what is available. The vinegar acts as a preservative and draws out the plants' components.

Vinegar itself is helpful for digestion and aids calcium absorption. This vinegar can be used to flavor vegetables and salads or used in a salad dressing together with oil and low-sodium tamari (soy sauce).

Hormones on the Rocks

A number of alcoholic drinks contain phytoestrogens. Drinks made with grains, including barley, rice, and corn, are likely to be estrogenic, as are those with added hops, aniseed, and other herbs.

Studies have demonstrated that isoflavones in bourbon can stimulate the uteri of rats that have had their ovaries removed; luteinizing hormone is lowered and the isoflavones can interact with estrogen receptors.[46] Bourbon with the alcohol removed at a dose equivalent to 4 ounces a day for twenty days changes the hormone status of postmenopausal women.[47]

Researchers suggest that phytoestrogens in alcohol may be responsible for feminization (such as breast development), which, along with cirrhosis of the liver, occurs in some male alcoholics. Female alcoholics have a higher risk of breast cancer, as they may be getting excess phytoestrogens. On the other hand, moderate alcohol consumption is linked to reduced cardiovascular disease.

Excessive alcohol is not appropriate menopause therapy, but if you like a drink, one serving a day may provide a little relief from both stress and menopausal symptoms. Alcoholic drinks that contain phytoestrogens include the following:

- Bourbon (isoflavones)
- Beer (isoflavones and hops)
- Red wine (resveratrol)
- Pernod and ouzo (estrogenic oil in aniseed)

Other drinks such as whiskey may contain estrogenic substances because they are produced from grains; other additional hormonal compounds may develop during fermentation, aging, and storage.

SAMPLE MENUS FOR REDUCING MENOPAUSAL SYMPTOMS

The following menus suggest ways to get a therapeutic level of phytoestrogenic foods in your diet to reduce menopausal symptoms.

Summer

Breakfast

Whole-grain cereal plus eight almonds served with soy yogurt or soy milk and fresh or frozen berries

or

Soy smoothie plus one to two soy cookies later for midmorning snack

Lunch

Whole-grain rye bread spread with miso plus mung bean sprouts, avocado, tomato, and other salad greens plus a piece of fruit

or

Cold whole-grain rice mixed with pumpkin seeds or cashews together with grated vegetables and finely chopped parsley and other herbs

Dinner

Chilled melon slices

Grilled fish with grilled potatoes, vegetables, or salad (flavor the vegetables with herbal vinegar and low-sodium tamari)

Rice cakes with soy cheese (for dessert)

Winter

Breakfast

Soy menopause porridge (see page 85)
or
Buckwheat, millet flakes, ground flaxseed, and raisin porridge

Lunch

Lentil, barley, and vegetable soup or curry, flavored with miso
or
Whole-grain bread grilled with soy cheese and tomato

Dinner

Corn on the cob
Soy and linseed burger served with vegetables
or
Lean beef and vegetable stir-fry, including bean sprouts

These sample menus are given to show how easy it is to get a high phytoestrogen diet. Once your menopausal symptoms have passed, reduce the quantities of phytoestrogenic foods. A truly healthy diet is varied, so avoid eating the same foods every day. Phytoestrogens are better absorbed and more effective therapeutically in smaller quantities at intervals rather than in one very large daily serving. Foods such as fruit or rice cakes can be used as snacks. In addition, always ensure an adequate fluid intake.

Men and Phytoestrogens

Don't think that you have to work out separate menus for yourself and your partner. Although men do not require the same high level of phytoestrogens that menopausal women may need, all the recommended foods in this chapter are suitable for men. Japan and some other Asian countries have a low death rate from prostate cancer compared with European countries.

When Japanese people adopt Western diets and lifestyles, they develop Western levels of cancer. In Japan, the intake of soy products averages about 39 grams daily, but many people have a much higher intake as well as a diet relatively low in fat and animal protein. Rural Finnish men who have a high intake of rye and berries also have a low incidence of prostate cancer. Seventh Day Adventist men who have a high intake of beans, lentils, peas, and dried fruit also have a decreased prostate cancer risk.

Over thirty studies support the prostate cancer preventive effect of phytoestrogens such as isoflavones and lignans.[48]

FOOD SUPPLEMENTS

Most developed countries now manufacture concentrated or isolated isoflavones, mainly combinations of genistein, daidzein, biochanin-A, and formononetin. These products are usually sold in the form of powders and tablets. In my opinion there is no substitute for healthy food, but these supplements may help you while you are learning to have a diet rich in phytoestrogens or as a dietary addition if you have severe menopausal symptoms.

Some supplements, however, are overpriced, especially some tablet products. Read the labels carefully to find the quantity of isoflavones in the product. It is usually more economical to buy in powder form.

A dosage of 20 milligrams of isoflavones daily may help very mild menopausal symptoms, but for severe flushing you may need 50 milligrams three times daily. If you take 150 milligrams once daily, your body may not be able to absorb that quantity at one time, so I suggest spreading out the daily intake. If this very high intake does not reduce your symptoms within three months, you need to look at other options.

No one has established an "official" dosage or done long-term studies on isoflavones as a treatment or preventive for osteoporosis, heart disease, and cancer. In the meantime I suggest about 50 milligrams daily to most patients, which can easily be obtained from the diet. This 50 milligram dosage is probably the quantity required as a maintenance preventive dose, assuming you have a healthy, varied diet and lifestyle.

Table 3.3 lists the approximate isoflavone content of a few common soy foods.

It is quite easy to get a therapeutic dose of 50 milligrams a day with normal dietary servings. Remember also that other healthful foods also contain phytoestrogens and other beneficial compounds.

TABLE 3.3 Isoflavone Content of Soy Foods	
Food	*Approximate Isoflavone Content*
1 cup soy milk	40 mg
½ cup tofu or tempeh	40 mg
½ cup cooked soybeans	35 mg
½ cup cooked textured vegetable protein	35 mg
1 ounce soy nuts	35 mg

From the available evidence, the majority of menopausal and post-menopausal women would benefit more by eating the foods recommended in this chapter than by taking hormone pills. Naturally occurring plant estrogens in edible foods are generally part of what could be described as a nutrient-rich, high-fiber diet that protects against a number of diseases. Of course, you should be doing other things to prevent health problems: consuming a varied diet with foods in as natural a state as possible, being physically active, relaxing, learning how to enjoy your life without harmful excesses, and being a noble but nonfanatical human being.

No one has evaluated the effect of combining phytoestrogens with hormone replacement therapy scientifically, but I suggest that eating phytoestrogenic foods in reasonable quantities may help balance your estrogens. Taking concentrated isoflavone supplements, however, would undoubtedly interfere with HRT and Tamoxifen, so it makes sense to avoid taking two completely different medications at the same time.

If you have severe flushing or other symptoms that are not alleviated by a phytoestrogen-rich diet or isoflavone supplements, my experience is that herbal formulas are often helpful. They deal with the problem from other perspectives, such as counteracting stress, lowering heat, relaxing blood vessels, and calming the nervous system.

CHAPTER FOUR

Sprouts and Vegelets:
Super Menopause Foods

I have given sprouts and young plants (vegelets) a separate chapter because they belong to a class of their own. They are highly recommended foods for the menopausal transition, particularly for women who are experiencing symptoms.

Plants have been studied for their estrogenic content at the first stages of growth. At the "seedling" stage, when the plants are about 2 to 3 inches tall, the levels of phytoestrogens are considerably higher than that found in the seeds. Plants undergo major transformations when they first begin to grow (a process called germination). In addition to their advantageous hormonal effects for menopausal women, sprouts and vegelets have nutritional qualities that make them very beneficial.

The seed of a plant is a concentrated food storage unit; it contains everything that the emerging baby plant will need for its first few days of life. When the seed is soaked in water, the outer covering is softened and the process of growing or germination begins. The root is the first part to emerge from the seed.

The young root shoot generally forms the main part of a sprout. Asian sprouting methods in particular carry out the process in a dark environment, and sometimes this pale young root shoot may be the only part eaten. The idea behind dark sprouting conditions is that it mimics what would be happening below ground level in normal plant growth; by placing sprouts in the light, you encourage growth of the green leaf shoot, that is, the normal aboveground growth. For instance, when you buy alfalfa sprouts, you get a combination of root and leaf shoot plus the residue of the seed.

Sprouting does not require fertilizers because the nutrients are supplied by the seed itself and plant growth is stimulated by the plant's own hormones.

As an approximate guide, most sprouts are ready for use in three days, although wheat sprouts are best used within two days of sprouting, before they get "stringy." The best time for soybean sprouts is about eight days, and for most other legumes it is four to five days.

There are many advantages of sprouted seeds.

- They are a good source of beneficial phytoestrogens.
- They are not limited by seasonal availability.
- Soil and sunlight are not necessary.
- They are economical in comparison with most vegetables, especially if you sprout your own.
- Dried seeds can be stored for an extended period and then turned into fresh vegetables within a week. With water, heating, and light, sprouting can be done indoors in cold regions.
- They are rich in nutrients but low in calories. The changes that take place during germination are nutritionally beneficial.
- The yield is relatively high.
- Although sprouts by themselves are a bit boring, they can be used to introduce more variety into the diet. For nonconverts, the taste is usually enhanced when they are slightly cooked or heated (with the exception of alfalfa).
- Watching plants develop may encourage you and your family to grow and eat your own vegetables.
- No weeding or peeling is required.

- There is no necessity for chemicals, synthetic growth hormones, or added plant nutrients.

In some regions of the world, the sprouted seeds are dried and turned into a type of flour that is not only richer in a number of nutrients than the seed but is often more digestible. It is surprising that dried legume-sprout flour has not been commercialized.

Later in this chapter, I give details about making your own sprouts, because people who live in rural areas may not be able to buy them or they are not readily available in many varieties. If you buy sprouts, always look at the bottom of the container to see if they are green or pale, not soggy and brownish in the middle and bottom.

PHYTOESTROGENIC CONTENT OF SPROUTS

Because hormones are needed to stimulate the growth of plants, it seems reasonable that all sprouts would be a relatively rich source of phytoestrogens, and I recommend them highly as a treatment for menopausal symptoms (see table 4.1). Detailed figures are not available for other legumes and grains, but it is known that mung bean, alfalfa, and red clover sprouts contain a higher level of phytoestrogens than the seeds (see table 4.2).

TABLE 4.1 Soy Seed and Sprout Comparison			
Germination time in days	Soy phytoestrogen content (mg/kg) dry		
	Daidzein	Genistein	Coumestrol
0	723.2	939.2	2.0
5	932.5	958.8	39.7
9	1,763.2	1,032.2	128.1

Source: G. Wang et al., "A Simplified HPLC Method for the Determination of Phytoestrogens in Soybean and Its Processed Products," Journal of Agriculture and Food Chemistry 38 (1990): 188.

TABLE 4.2 **Mung Bean Seed and Sprout Comparison**

	Genistein	Daidzein
	(mg/100 g)	
Mung bean seeds	365	9.7
Mung bean sprouts	1,902	745.0

Source: H. Aldercreutz and W. Mazur, "Phytoestrogens and Western Diseases," *Annals of Medicine* 29 (1997): 99.

NUTRIENT CONTENT OF SPROUTS

Over 400 years ago, Western explorers discovered that sprouted legumes and seeds contained antiberiberi and antiscurvy nutrients. In the early twentieth century, it was noted that about a teaspoon of germinated peas or lentils was equivalent in vitamin content to around 2 tablespoons of carrots or ½ teaspoon of lemon or orange juice. In the early 1900s, in a military hospital, sick soldiers were fed about ¾ cup of germinated beans each day, and 70 percent were cured of scurvy (vitamin C deficiency) within four weeks, compared with the 54 percent of those fed the same quantity of fresh lemon juice. During the Indian famine of the 1930s, it was found that scurvy in children was cured and prevented by about 3 tablespoons of germinated grain twice weekly.

The examples in table 4.3 show that essential nutrients are increased when seeds are sprouted. Note, however, that there are wide variations in both seed and sprout nutrients according to the species of plant, the health of the seed, temperatures, degree of light, composition of the soaking and rinsing water, growing time, moisture content, handling, and storage.

Vitamins

Vitamin C The most important nutritional change brought on by sprouting is the plant's own production of vitamin C (ascorbic acid). This knowledge could be crucial in circumstances where grain or legume seeds

TABLE 4.3 Nutrient Content of Seeds Compared with Young Sprouts (percent, based on dry weight)

	Lentils		Mung beans		Peas		Soybeans		Alfalfa		Wheat	
	Seed	*Sprout*	*Seed*	*Sprout*	*Seed*	*Sprout*	*Seed*	*Sprout*	*Seed*	*Sprout*	*Seed*	*Sprout*
Protein	27.2	39.7	25.9	39.8	24.0	38.2	39.6	43.9	37.2	45.3	11.5	13.7
Vitamin C	0.0	234.6	0.0	105.1	0.0	140.7	0.0	172.8	0.0	228.9	0.0	5.1
Niacin	2.4	7.2	2.1	9.3	2.9	6.6	3.3	5.7	1.9	7.4	4.1	5.7
Zinc	4.8	7.1	3.4	4.9	2.5	4.4	3.9	5.9	6.9	8.6	2.9	3.2

Source: R. H. Matthews (ed.), *Legumes: Chemistry, Technology, and Human Nutrition* (New York: Marcel Dekker, 1989).

are the only food available, because most dry, nongerminated food seeds contain little or none of this vitamin. Although sprouts may be cultivated in the dark, those grown in the light make more vitamin C.

Water-Soluble B Vitamins   Most water-soluble B vitamins are increased significantly by sprouting. At the very least, the sprout has about the same content as the seed.

Vitamin A and Carotene   Evidence shows that the carotene content of grains and legumes can be more than doubled during germination. (Carotene is converted in your body to a usable form of vitamin A.)

Some young sprouts such as alfalfa, radish, and cress compare favorably with many vegetables in carotene content; radish sprouts are also very high in vitamin C: 316 milligrams per 100 grams.[1]

Vitamin E   An early study showed that in seven legumes and three grains, vitamin E increased by around 25 percent compared with the seeds after four days sprouting.[2]

Vitamin K   From the few tests that have been carried out, mainly on legumes, vitamin K may increase by 13 to 85 percent after four days sprouting and even more if continued growth is allowed.

Minerals

The question of how much of each mineral you absorb is as important as the actual quantity in the food. Seeds of all types are relatively high in phytate, a substance that may slightly reduce mineral absorption. During sprouting, however, the plant's metabolism is such that phytate levels are markedly reduced, resulting in improved absorption of the calcium, iron, and zinc present in the sprouts.

When distilled water has been used for soaking and rinsing sprouts, the minerals may be leached from them into the water and mineral losses may be as high as 40 percent. Conversely, a Chinese study found a large increase in the calcium content of soaked mung bean sprouts, which was attributed to the high mineral content of the water being used ("hard" water).

Protein and Fats

Nearly all studies indicate that protein is increased during the process of sprouting. During soaking and germination, changes take place in the plant's fat chemistry. Three days' germination of alfalfa, lentils, mung, and soybeans decreased fat content by 62, 39, 31, and 55 percent, respectively. Legumes in the diet generally lower blood fats, including cholesterol.

P. L. Finney wrote that the common use of sprouts in the diets of Asian people rests on a sound nutritional base and should be introduced on a wide scale among other people. After conducting a number of scientific studies himself and reviewing 313 research papers, he concluded that "carefully controlled, optimal germination of edible cereals and legumes is capable of significantly alleviating today's food problems and avoiding tomorrow's food needs."[3]

Enzymes

A significant change occurs in the enzymatic activity of germinating seeds; most enzymes reach maximum activity between two and six days of sprouting. The enzyme amylase is present in high quantities because starch is being broken down, which explains why young sprouts taste sweetish and are more digestible than seeds and grains. Because this enzyme is found in humans only after the age of six months, blended grain sprouts may be a better "weaning food" than cereal grains.

Antinutrients in Legumes

Legumes are basically plants that produce pods, such as peas and beans. They are generally acknowledged as being beneficial in human nutrition, and they contain phytoestrogens. They also contain two groups of substances that are classed as antinutrients, however, because if they are eaten raw or insufficiently cooked they interfere with digestion and absorption. Sprouting reduces these disadvantages.

Oligosaccharides (Raffinose, Stachyose, and Verbascose) Oligosaccharides are carbohydrates that are nondigestible by humans and that have to be broken down by bacterial activity, which produces carbon dioxide and hydrogen, that is, the main components of gastrointestinal gas. These particular carbohydrates are converted to digestible starches by soaking, germination, and cooking; hence, I recommend that legume sprouts be cooked. Some of these carbohydrates, however, act as substrates (building blocks) for the beneficial bacteria in your intestines.

Antitrypsin Factor Raw legumes contain a factor that interferes with the enzyme trypsin, which is necessary for the digestion of protein. Therefore, don't eat raw legumes (although a few green peas would not cause any problems). Alfalfa and mung bean sprouts contain only minimal quantities of these antinutrients, and so these sprouts may be eaten raw. Cooking, however, makes legume sprouts more digestible,[4] and I think cooking makes them tastier. There's a good side effect of antitrypsin: it has cancer-preventive activity.

Sprouts of large or very hard beans, such as soybeans, are best when lightly cooked for seven to ten minutes; I like them steamed, cooled, and in salads. Other bean sprouts can be simply added to stir-fries, casseroles, or soups just before serving so that they are heated through to the center. You can also steam legume sprouts and use them cold in salads.

MAKING YOUR OWN SPROUTS

All commercial horticultural seeds, unless specifically stated otherwise, are treated with fungicides or other chemicals, so you must use seeds sold either as food or specifically for sprouting. The basic rule is to use only known edible foods. The shoots and leaves of some edible foods—including tomato, pepper, eggplant, potato, and rhubarb—are highly poisonous, however, so their seeds are never used for sprouting. In addition, sorghum sprouts contain naturally occurring cyanide, and loupini (lupin) seeds contain toxic quantities of a bitter-tasting alkaloid that is not destroyed by cooking or sprouting.

I usually begin by soaking the seeds overnight, although those that become wrinkly, such as soybeans, are best with a short soaking time, more rinsing, and very thorough draining. Although most sprouts will keep quite well in the refrigerator for many days, it is best to use them within a few days. Some of the nutrients start to diminish with long storage, and they can develop fungi or harmful bugs if they are left too long.

Some books tell you that growing sprouts is foolproof, quick, and easy, but I don't find it all that easy. Once you develop a routine and find out what suits your taste and environment, however, it is not too time consuming, can save you money, and can improve your health.

I suggest that you use a variety of sprouts from the list below and in table 4.4. Owing to the estrogen content of most sprouts, consuming large quantities may not be advisable for men or young children.

How Much Should You Eat?

For menopausal women, with severe flushing, 1 cup of sprouts daily would be a therapeutic intake. You may not be able to eat this much, however, because sprouts need to be mixed with other foods unless you want to have, say, mung or soybean sprouts steamed and cooled as a snack. For long-term use, I suggest about ½ cup every second day, with somewhat less for men and proportionately less for children.

Seeds Suitable for Sprouting

Seeds suitable for sprouting include alfalfa, aniseed, barley, beans, buckwheat, cabbage, caraway, celery, chickpeas, collard, corn, cress, dill, fennel, fenugreek, kale, lentils, mustard, oats, peas, radish, red clover, turnip, and wheat. These seeds are all dried, whole, chemical free, and unprocessed. Table 9 lists general guidelines for sprouting seeds.

Some Specific Sprouting Methods

The following are a few of the ways in which you can produce your own sprouts; in addition, a number of different types of commercial, plastic sprouters are on the market and usually include instructions. Some people

TABLE 4.4 Guidelines for Sprouting Seeds

Aniseed, caraway, dill, and fennel	I use these combined with other sprouts. In combinations, it's better to mix seeds that are more or less the same size.
Barley, oats, rice, and wheat	Only a few days' sprouting is recommended. They are ideal cooked in bread or savory scones, as thickening for soups or casseroles, or in sandwiches.
Beans	Smaller beans are easier to sprout than larger beans. Mung beans are my favorite because they are not "temperamental" and are the only sprouted beans that don't require cooking; adzuki are the next best choice, followed by borlotti and navy beans. Soybeans are difficult to sprout; I find my homemade soy sprouts do not get shoots as long as those found in grocery stores, but they are worth the effort because they are quite tasty and are absolutely the best source of phytoestrogens. Broad, lima, and kidney beans are also difficult to sprout, as are chickpeas. These large, hard legume seeds generally require a shorter soaking time, warmer temperatures, more frequent rinsing, good drainage, and plenty of air, or they become moldy and smelly and are inedible.
Cabbage family	All the plants in this family may be sprouted, including cabbage, collard, kale, mustard, radish, and turnip. Some are strong and spicy, so I usually mix them in with alfalfa.
Corn	The raw sprouts make very sweet, chewy snacks.

You can sprout many other seeds, but some of them, such as sunflower, either do not taste as nice as the seed itself or are too much trouble to sprout. Herbs such as coriander and tarragon are too strong and unpalatable for sprouting.

use wet muslin (lightweight cloth with airholes) supported by wire frames; others use plastic containers with drainage and airholes pushed through them. If you look in your kitchen cupboards, you will find something you can use or adapt.

Alfalfa Soak 2 to 3 tablespoons of seeds overnight in a large jar (at least 2-pint capacity) of tepid water.

Around the top of the jar use something like nylon netting affixed with a thick rubber band; I find that cheesecloth tends to prevent aeration and may cause the seeds to go moldy.

The next day, strain out the soaking water, rinse the seeds with tepid water, strain them thoroughly, and if possible leave the jar upside down at a 45-degree angle so that none of the seeds becomes soggy.

Repeat the rinsing and straining procedure night and morning for about three to six days, keeping the jar in a light, warm position once the sprouts begin to grow if you want green, leafy growth.

Both seeds and new growth are fairly delicate, so don't subject them to direct sunlight.

They are usually harvested when they are about 1½ inches long.

Some people give the sprouts a vigorous rinsing at the end of the sprouting time so that the brownish outside part of the seed floats to the surface and can be washed off. (I don't do this rinse.) The sprouts are then thoroughly drained and ready for eating. Store them in the refrigerator, preferably in a fairly low container, and they will continue to sprout slowly.

Thoroughly clean and dry all equipment between batches.

Although alfalfa sprouts are commonly used in sandwiches and salads, you can chop and mash them into cottage cheese or use them as a thickening agent in cooked dishes simply by stirring them in just before serving.

Mung Beans Mung beans are worth mentioning separately because they are the easiest to sprout even if you sometimes forget to rinse them or if the temperature is low.

Mung beans can be prepared in the same way as alfalfa, but here is a different method:

- Wash the beans first and soak them overnight in a jar of tepid water.
- In the morning place them in a flat plastic tray that has drainage holes. They will need something to drain onto. (I use an old plastic breakfast tray.)
- Rinse twice daily and discard the water that has drained onto the tray.
- Mung beans are best harvested when they are between 1 to 3 inches long.

I prefer them grown in darkish conditions, which keeps the root shoot pale and vigorous. If you want to keep them outdoors, you will need to cover them to keep them clean and not exposed to too much light. Just don't forget about them if they're not in the kitchen.

An alternate method is to put the seeds onto nylon netting that is resting in a tray of moist vermiculite and give them a spray of water daily to keep the vermiculite moist. When they are ready for harvesting, just lift them up with the netting and then rinse and drain them. Any bits of vermiculite sticking to the netting will be washed off.

All sprouts should be stored in the refrigerator.

Mung bean sprouts don't have to be cooked, but they are excellent as a thickening agent in soups and casseroles.

Wheat   I use biodynamic wheat and find that it sprouts quickly and easily, even under adverse or cold conditions. After overnight soaking, sprouting should be allowed to continue for a maximum of three days (less in warm weather). If you let the root grow more than ¼ inch, it becomes stringy. The sprouts are somewhat chewy but are delicious cold, lightly cooked, or in homemade bread or savory cookies. Both methods given above also work quite well for wheat.

Cress and Mustard   Cress and mustard seeds are best not soaked because they tend to be sticky. Mustard in particular develops a furry root system, so don't discard the sprouts thinking that they have gone moldy.

My system for these and other small seeds is to place them outside in a shady place in a large plastic seedling tray lined with weed-control mat and filled with about an inch of vermiculite. I cover the vermiculite with fine nylon netting, and after placing the seeds on the vermiculite I cover the trays with shadecloth for protection while allowing for air movement. I give them a fine water spray one to three times daily to keep them moist and harvest them when they are about 1 inch high. I usually just pull them out in little clumps as required, but you need to wash the cloth or netting after each batch.

This method of sprouting is good for seeds that have a very husky outer covering, such as buckwheat, as it saves rinsing off the hulls. The vermiculite should be dried in the sun between batches.

Why Seeds Don't Germinate

Seeds may not germinate for a number of reasons, as follows:

- Sometimes the seeds are damaged or too old.
- Processed seeds will not grow. Make sure that you use intact seeds, that is, those with their outer coat still on. Ask if the particular seeds you want are suitable for sprouting.
- Many seeds from hybridized (manipulated) plants are sterile. That's how the companies make money; the seeds developed by the plant itself will not grow and you have to buy them from the company for each crop. In other words, collecting seeds yourself may not work.
- The temperature may be inappropriate for the particular plant species. For example, peas won't develop if it is too hot and soybeans won't sprout if it is too cold. I use a special "grow light," sold by plant nurseries, which makes my sprouting area warmer in winter.
- The amount of moisture may be unsuitable: excess water will cause rotting, whereas lack of water prevents growth.
- If the seeds are crammed too closely together, they will not get the amount of oxygen and water sufficient for growth.

Don't be discouraged if you have a few failures when you are learning, but if a batch goes "off," you should scald the equipment before reusing it.

Optimum Sprouting Conditions

It is not possible to be precise about optimum sprouting because there are so many plants and so many variations of the same plant. Most seeds, if conditions are ideal, will be ready to eat as sprouts from two to six days after soaking. A temperature around 77°F generally works best for most of my sprouts, but your kitchen may be much colder or warmer than conditions outside. Experimentally, germination of wheat can occur from 37°F to 107°F, so you can see that there is a wide range for some seeds. In very cold conditions, however, growth of some seeds may be too slow to produce edible sprouts, and in very high temperatures, fungal growth may spoil the sprouts. Many seeds will not germinate in extremes of temperature.

The overall aims are to keep seeds moist but not soggy, to ensure that they have a good air supply, and to keep the equipment very clean.

Adverse Reactions to Sprouts

Alfalfa, and to a lesser extent other legumes, contains a compound called canavanine that is destroyed by cooking but not by sprouting. This compound has been implicated in a few cases worldwide of lupus (systemic lupus erythematosus), an autoimmune arthritic disorder somewhat similar to rheumatoid arthritis. This same compound, however, is now considered to be an active anticancer agent.[5] If you develop lupus, stop eating alfalfa and legume sprouts and make sure all legume foods are well cooked. Because rare adverse reactions occur in susceptible people, this advice does not mean that everyone should avoid the foods in question; otherwise, there would be nothing in the world we could eat.

There have been a few reports of sprouts being contaminated with harmful microorganisms (bugs). Virtually all fresh and cooked foods can contain these if they are not handled and stored correctly. Sprouts should be used within a week of sprouting, stored in the refrigerator without being packed closely together so that they can continue to grow slowly. Don't use them if they are soggy, smelly, or moldy.

VEGELETS (MINI VEGETABLES)

Vegelets, as I like to call them, are more like giant sprouts than vegetables. If nothing else, they provide a good way of using up seeds or growing your own food in confined spaces. The big advantages (compared with growing vegetables) are that you get a quick crop and, of course, the satisfaction of growing your own food.

Snow Peas

Snow peas are my favorite vegelet. If you grow them into vegetables you may be disappointed, because you have to wait a long time for them to mature and you don't get many pods per plant, which explains why they are expensive to buy.

My method is to grow them outside in filtered sun, using shallow polystyrene boxes or plastic trays (about 12 inches square) with about 1½ inches of light soil that is rich in composted organic matter or potting mix. (The containers must have drainage or airholes at the bottom.)

I sprinkle the seeds evenly over the soil, cover them with about ¾ inch of potting mix, water thoroughly, and then don't apply any more water until the shoots appear.

Once the shoots appear, I water them lightly once a day.

If you harvest the aboveground growth when it is about 4 to 5 inches high, cutting it above the lowest leaf shoot, within a week or so you will get a second and even a third crop. This method is very economical, because you can get up to fifteen boxes or up to forty-five crops from about 1 pound of seeds.

These greens have a delicious, pea flavor. Chop them into salads or sandwiches or add them to stir-fries and other cooked dishes just before serving so that they are heated through.

I also grow snow peas inside, using perlite or vermiculite instead of soil and keeping them under a special "grow light." Perlite and vermiculite don't contain any nutrients but simply support the plant and store water, so you need to use a liquid fertilizer or hydroponic fluid if you want successive crops from the one batch of seeds. You can also grow vegelets in the garden, but don't grow too many at one time.

Wheat Grass

I grow wheat grass like snow pea vegelets. When it is 4 inches high, I chop it off with a scissors just above the soil level. The first crop is surprisingly sweet. Harvesting in this way produces a number of crops, because wheat grass regrows after cutting. It is somewhat "grassy" tasting but quite pleasant. Use it liberally, chopped up finely like chives in salads or in cooked meals. Sometimes I just munch on a handful, and a little wheat grass is quite pleasant in carrot or other juices.

I could not find any recent, reliable nutritional information for wheat grass, although I presume that it is extremely high in chlorophyll, carotenoids, and vitamin K.

Barley

Barley grown like wheat grass tastes quite "grassy," but it is not noticeable when it is finely chopped and mixed into a salad. Barley is one of the best grains for lowering cholesterol and improving glucose metabolism. It germinates very easily in cooler conditions.

According to information supplied by a manufacturer of a barley leaf product and from tests done by the Resource Research Association, Japan, the juice from young barley leaves contains eleven times more calcium than cow's milk, nearly five times the iron content of spinach, nearly seven times the vitamin C in oranges, and four times the vitamin B_I in whole wheat flour! Young barley leaves would undoubtedly be very rich in carotenoids, plant hormones of various kinds, and would contain glycosyl-isovitexin (a powerful antioxidant) and other ingredients that reduce blood stickiness. In addition, in common with all dark green edible plants, barley leaves are rich in chlorophyll, which is one of nature's "cleansers" as well as a helper in carrying oxygen within your body.

Barley greens are available commercially as drinks and powders. These products have been found to lower cholesterol, improve endurance, and provide other health advantages.

Other Advantages of Vegelets

By using my basic vegelet system, I have grown and eaten bean greens, buckwheat, radicchio (a bitter vegetable popular with Italians), lettuce, salad rocket, Italian parsley, fennel, carrot tops, mustard, silver beet, bok choy and other Asian vegetables, kale, collard, and most plants in the cabbage family. Some plants are not suitable for cultivation as vegelets; these plants are listed under sprouts.

My system provides a wide variety of vegetable greens over a short time, with all their associated nutritional and hormonal advantages. There is no need to use artificial fertilizers or pesticides. If necessary, you can rig up a shelter with shadecloth to protect the little plants from slugs, snails, and leaf-eating insects.

Hormones are present in vegelets as well as in sprouts; seedlings of green beans have been shown to contain tiny amounts of estrone and estradiol. Phytosterols (hormone-like compounds) are known to be high in young green plants, and they have estrogenic effects in animals.[6] Some types of phytosterols improve human immune function,[7] and some animal studies show that they have the potential to inhibit tumor formation. As mentioned in chapter 3, they can also reduce menopausal symptoms and lower cholesterol.

Because the world's population is increasing dramatically and the amount of arable land per person is proportionately decreasing, it's not unrealistic to suggest that there will come a time when we must use the available agricultural land for growing seeds and actually producing food in the areas inside and around our houses.

As you can see, there are many health and environmental advantages of growing sprouts and vegelets and remarkably few disadvantages. And, it's fun.

CHAPTER FIVE

Menopause Herbs and Other Natural Remedies

*F*oods with beneficial estrogenic effects are listed and explained in chapters 3 and 4. If you include these foods in your diet, menopause symptoms may be relieved and some degenerative diseases may be prevented.

Remember, however, that with menopause—as with most health problems—there are mild symptoms that require either no treatment or simply improvements you can make yourself, there are other instances where a consultation with a professional natural therapist is appropriate, and there are severe or complicated cases that require a medical diagnosis and treatment. There are also confounding factors. For instance, menopause symptoms can coincide with other problems. Or, what appear to be hormonal symptoms may have another cause; for example, sweating and heat may be due to fever, infection, or, in rare cases, a brain tumor. Find the cause of any health problem as far as possible.

HERBS WITH ESTROGEN-LIKE ACTIVITY

Many estrogenic plants have been "tested" for centuries on millions of women with menstrual problems, with remarkably few adverse reactions. I have observed their benefits in my clinic for two decades. Compared with hormone replacement therapy, which increases the risk of cancer and numerous other problems, medicinal herbs offer a number of good side effects because they contain many components. When used appropriately, herbs have remarkably few adverse reactions (in my experience, about 1 person in 500).

Medicinal herbs in the form of herbal teas are not very strong. Liquid extracts, powders, and some tablets and capsules, however, are quite concentrated, so you need to follow the dosages on the labels of any products you buy. If you have severe symptoms, there is no reason why you can't have foods containing phytoestrogens, plus one or two herbal remedies in a concentrated form; a few cups of herbal teas; a regular, generous use of culinary herbs; and even a serving of an alcoholic drink.

Plants contain hundreds of different constituents; consequently, they have a variety of effects in your body. There is not one plant in the world that doesn't contain some toxic compounds (to protect the plant itself). In edible foods and medicinal herbs, these compounds are more than offset by the benefits, and your body has a system of enzymes that can handle the tiny amounts of naturally occurring toxins.

The most important menopause herbs along with details to help you choose what suits you, based on your menopausal symptoms and on any other coexisting problems, are listed in this chapter. Celery seeds, for example, contain phytoestrogens and also have antiarthritic and diuretic properties, so this herb would be an appropriate remedy if you have menopausal symptoms along with fluid retention and joint problems.

Medicinal herbs will not give as much phytoestrogens as you would get in the diet, but it is the total therapeutic properties of an herb that provide the most benefit. My clinical experience is that a number of herbs in a formula provides a better result than a single herb. Furthermore, a better therapeutic effect for many women results from two formulas: tonic herbs in the morning and relaxant herbs in the evening. Although it might not seem holistic, this approach works for many women in my clinic who complain of fatigue during the day and who also have difficulty getting adequate or refreshing sleep.

IMPORTANT MENOPAUSAL HERBS

For all the herbs listed in table 5.1, take the label dosage. A number of these herbs may be available in tablet form, but in most cases you will need to visit an herbalist to get a formula that is most appropriate for you.

Generally, you should get marked relief of menopause symptoms within twelve weeks.

TABLE 5.1 **Important Menopause Herbs**

Phytoestrogenic Herb	*Secondary Therapeutic Effects*
Morning formula (using liquid extracts; might include up to eight of the following):	
Alfalfa	Cholesterol lowering; general tonic
Aniseed	Antiflatulent; helpful for coughs
Astragalus	Immune and general tonic
Black cohosh	Relaxant for joints, muscles, blood vessels
Licorice	Anti-inflammatory; general tonic
Paeonia	May reduce fibrocystic breast disease
Other herbs that are not phytoestrogenic but may be helpful:	
Asian and Siberian ginseng	Supports physical and mental stresses
St. John's wort	Antidepressant; immune tonic
Gotu kola	Nerve and memory aid; antiarthritic; hair tonic
Saw palmetto	Urinary tract toner
Tribulus terrestris	Indian restorative herb

(continued overleaf)

TABLE 5.1 *(continued)*

Phytoestrogenic Herb	Secondary Therapeutic Effects
Evening formula (using liquid extracts; might include up to six of the following):	
Corn silk	Antifungal; anti-inflammatory; soothes bladder
Fennel	Antiflatulent
Hops	Sedative; liver and digestive aid
Red clover	Relaxant; also used for coughs and skin problems
Sage	Antiseptic; antisweating; memory aid
Shepherd's purse	Urinary tract healer and antiseptic
Other herbs that are not phytoestrogenic but may be helpful:	
Hawthorn	Antioxidant; helps blood vessels; lowers blood pressure
Schisandra	Liver tonic; may reduce sweating
Valerian	Sedative; digestive aid

Dosage guidelines

Morning formula:	5 to 10 ml after breakfast
Evening formula:	2½ to 5 ml after dinner and 2½ to 5 ml before bedtime

To cover the taste, I recommend either black grape juice or a berry juice; these juices may also have some slight estrogenic effect as well as being excellent antioxidants. Don't have too much fluid with the evening formula, however, because your bladder may not cope.

Hops (*Humulus lupulus*)

My own laboratory tests and an early German study showed that hops is by far the most estrogenic of all plants. It was noticed that when girls harvested hops by hand, they experienced changes in their menstrual patterns; thus, scientists began to test for hormonal activity. Hops, however, is not a high-dose herb, so you do not get as much isoflavonic phytoestrogens as you do from eating soy foods. On the other hand, hops has some relevant therapeutic qualities.

Hops is a remedy for insomnia, and traditionally, hops pillows were used for sleeping. A European medical study showed that hops extract or a strong tea helped sleep when added to a bath. These external treatments are not likely to be universally popular because the aroma is awful and may not be sufficiently camouflaged with lavender or some other pleasant-smelling plant.

Studies on rats showed that hops has sedative and sleep-inducing properties, has heat-lowering properties, and relaxes muscles and reflexes.[1] Another animal study showed that hops can help detoxify certain chemicals without making them harmful.

Hops is a very bitter-tasting herb, which is why it is added to beer. It is excellent for the digestion and has some antibiotic effects.

I recommend hops as an after-dinner remedy, either as a tea or in the form of a liquid extract, taking about twenty to forty drops in water or juice. It can also be part of a formula. Herbalists never prescribe hops to people who are depressed, and I never use it as a daytime remedy.

Red Clover (*Trifolium repens*)

It has been known since the 1940s that when sheep graze on clover they become infertile, and isoflavonic phytoestrogens are responsible for this effect. The relatively small amounts that humans would get in a serving of sprouts, tea, tablets, or liquid extracts would not be anything like the quantity that sheep consume.

Red clover in herbal form has been prescribed traditionally for skin problems and coughs and as an anticancer remedy.[2]

I first began using red clover for hormonal problems in the early 1980s, and it seemed to be effective at a dose of around 5 grams of the herb per day, along with some dietary phytoestrogens. This broad approach gives a wide range of nutrients and therapeutic components compared with the approach of treating one problem with one compound. (Hardly any of my patients complain of only one problem.)

A few scientific studies have shown that a red clover tablet containing 40 to 160 milligrams of isoflavones is no more effective for reducing menopausal symptoms than placebo.[3] Some of the women on the sugar pill, however, were consuming phytoestrogens in their diet (as revealed in urine tests), so it may not have been a valid comparison. A red clover tablet containing 40 to 80 milligrams isoflavones, however, did increase the elasticity in the arteries in a study of twenty-seven postmenopausal women.[4]

I think that severe menopausal symptoms require about 150 milligrams isoflavones a day plus herbs or specific supplements for the multiplicity of problems that are likely to be present (as explained in chapter 1).

For women with severe menopausal symptoms, I recommend red clover in the form of sprouts because they are the richest source of phytoestrogens and because you get the benefits of the other components in the plant.

You can buy red clover tablets with standardized quantities of isoflavones in them, but study the labels. If the tablet contains only 40 milligrams isoflavones, that is the same quantity you could get in a cup of soy milk or a serving of sprouts. If you don't want to change your diet in line with chapters 3 and 4, you are better off buying a powder that contains isoflavones rather than an expensive but relatively weak tablet. Another option is to consult a practitioner to advise you about a natural therapies program that you can manage.

Licorice (*Glycyrrhiza glabra*)

Licorice contains over 334 known constituents, including phytoestrogens, phytosterols, flavonoids, and saponins. Some natural licorice may have the capacity to reduce the risk of breast cancer by changing estrogen metabolism in the body. Studies have shown that licorice can lower testosterone activity in the body; therefore, it may be appropriate if you have high levels of male hormones, which may be indicated by high libido or unwanted hair growth or determined by a blood test.

Licorice has a long history of use as a medicine for coughs, weakness, and inflammation and is supported by numerous research studies for its antiviral, antiulcer, anticholesterol, and liver detoxification effects. It is prescribed as an internal remedy for bronchitis and other coughs, gastritis (inflamed stomach), some types of gastric ulcers, fatigue, menopause symptoms, and many inflammatory and allergic conditions.

If you have fluid retention or a tendency to high blood pressure, do not use licorice internally in any form as it can deplete potassium in the body. Generally, it is considered that up to 3 grams a day of pure licorice root will not cause adverse effects.[5]

Licorice external cream is excellent for dry skin. It is often helpful for a dry vagina as long as the cream is made up in a quality ointment base. My recipe is as follows. Simmer 25 milliliters licorice liquid extract with 25 milliliters distilled water for three minutes. Cool, then mix the extract liquid into about 4 ounces (100 grams) of a thick, plain ointment base (a blender makes a smooth creamy product). Label with an expiration date of three months and store in the refrigerator. (It contains no preservatives because the alcohol has been simmered off.)

Licorice as an external remedy is also recommended for treating herpes.

Licorice confectionery is unlikely to have any therapeutic effects. In most countries, licorice candy contains very little licorice and a number of potentially harmful additives such as aniseed oil. One researcher has suggested that a safe daily dose of confectionery is about 5 grams.[6]

Black Cohosh (*Cimicifuga racemosa*)

A German study of menopausal women showed that a black cohosh product reduced luteinizing hormone levels (high levels of this hormone accompany menopausal flushing). The vaginal tissue of menopausal women was improved to the same degree as a pharmaceutical estrogen. Experiments in animals show that black cohosh can be taken up at estrogen binding sites in the body, which means that it has a similar effect as phytoestrogenic isoflavones.[7]

Eight studies have confirmed that black cohosh is effective for reducing menopause symptoms, and the herb is well-tolerated.[8] German doctors have been prescribing and studying black cohosh (mainly the brand Remifemin) as a treatment for menopause symptoms since the 1950s. Black cohosh contains formononetin, a phytoestrogen, as well as other hormone-like compounds.

In traditional American Indian medicine, black cohosh was used to treat rheumatism, to promote the flow of breast milk, and for infections and fevers. Early American medical herbalists prescribed black cohosh exten-sively; it was described as having special affinity for the female reproductive organs and effective for treating a wide range of female disorders.[9]

Although black cohosh has hormonal effects, reports confirm that it does not stimulate breast cancer cells, is nontoxic, and is suitable for women when pharmaceutical hormone therapy is contraindicated.[10]

Sage (*Salvia officinalis*)

In traditional herbal medicine, sage has been used to reduce sweating, to reduce breast milk after weaning, for infections, and as a gargle for sore throats. Generally, it is considered that the essential oils are the main thera-peutic component of sage. Tests have shown that sage is an excellent antiox-idant with some antibacterial and antifungal activity, which is why it was formerly used to help preserve foods.[11]

When I sent some sage for laboratory testing, results showed that sage contained small quantities of the phytoestrogens genistein, daidzein, and formononetin and phytosterols. Sage and alfalfa can be very helpful for reducing hot flashes and night sweats in menopausal women.

Danish researchers found that sage had effects on animal brain tissue, which may account for the reputation of this herb as a mild relaxant and brain tonic. A flavonoid in sage (apigenin) has antianxiety effects and pos-sibly estrogenic effects. In Germany, sage is used by physicians as an inter-nal remedy for indigestion and excessive perspiration.[12]

Sage contains some toxic compounds, but so do all plants. Generally, according to the Committee on Food Protection, we must continue to rely upon the remarkable capacity of the human body to deal promptly and effectively with small quantities of toxic materials.[13] Because of the very strong taste of sage as a culinary herb, it is unlikely that people would over-dose. In the form of medicinal extract or tablet, do not take more than the prescribed dose for three months without a break. Never use sage essential oil internally, and restrict external use of the oil to about ten drops. (I find it helpful rubbed into the scalp, but some people find it too strong.)

SAGE TEA

2 tablespoons finely chopped fresh leaves (or 1 tablespoon dried)

Soak overnight in 1 pint of tepid water and the juice of one lemon.

Strain in the morning, store in the refrigerator, and drink over the next one to two days.

To make it more palatable, drink cold sage tea with fruit or vegetable juice.

Asian Ginseng (*Panax ginseng*)

None of the ginsengs actually contains known phytoestrogens, but a number of reports suggest that Asian ginseng is helpful for menopause problems such as vaginal dryness.[14] Ginseng can reduce flushing and sweating in 80 to 90 percent of women. Studies with rats confirmed that Asian ginseng had a significant effect on basic nerve and hormone functions.[15]

Ginseng is one of the most scientifically researched herbs, with over 3,000 published studies, and there is abundant support for its antistress, tonic, and restorative properties as well as its disease- and infection-preventing capacity. Menopausal flushing is often worsened by stress, and this symptom is perhaps alleviated because of ginseng's antistress actions. Furthermore, the main therapeutic components in the herb are saponins, and their breakdown products may have hormonal effects along with the phytosterols (discussed in chapter 4). You can try Asian ginseng for yourself, but because it is a tonic herb, do not take it late in the day.

Most herbalists suggest not taking ginseng for longer than two or three months without a break.

Siberian ginseng is also an excellent antistress herb. I often use it in a menopause morning formula (see Table 10), although it can be used by itself.

Alfalfa (*Medicago sativa*)

Generally, sprouts are the best way to take alfalfa if you have severe menopausal problems. There is a limit to the quantity of sprouts you can reasonably consume in one day, however, because they're not particularly exciting to the taste buds. Alfalfa has similar hormone-balancing effects to soy (as explained in chapter 3), but it is not as strong because you consume less of it.

You can buy alfalfa tablets, tea, and liquid extracts that all contain phytoestrogenic isoflavones, and coumestrol. Three U.S. brands of alfalfa tablets were analyzed for their coumestrol content and were found to contain from 20 to 199 parts per million of this phytoestrogen.[16]

Traditional uses of alfalfa include as a lactation tonic for breast-feeding mothers, to reduce excess acidity in the stomach and joints, and for recuperation. Animal studies have shown that alfalfa lowers blood cholesterol and can reduce atherosclerosis.

Alfalfa is also an herb that stimulates rumors. Some authors warn people that coumestrol, and therefore alfalfa, can break down red blood cells in the body, but that happens only if these types of compounds are injected directly into the blood. Other authors suggest that alfalfa helps speed up the metabolism and therefore assists in weight loss, but I have not observed this effect in my clinic.

Aniseed and Fennel

For centuries, aniseed, fennel, and other herbs have been recognized for their hormonal effects. Anethole, an essential oil compound, contributes to the observed estrogenic effects of plants such as aniseed and fennel.[17]

These herbs are helpful for menopause symptoms; in addition, aniseed is useful for treating coughs, and fennel is classified as a remedy for stomach and various digestive problems. Herbal practitioners usually prescribe fennel and aniseed as concentrated liquid extracts, but they are also available in various tablet formulations.

The seeds and finely chopped fresh leaves of aniseed and fennel may be used in cooking, in salads, as herbal teas, and in herbal vinegars. They are used as flavoring agents in a number of foods and also in the production of alcoholic drinks such as gin, ouzo, and Pernod, but I don't recommend more than one serving daily of these strong drinks for therapeutic purposes.

Other foods and herbs in the Apiaceae family are also recommended for menopausal woman. They include celery (especially celery seed), parsley, caraway, carrots, cumin, coriander, dill, lovage, and parsnips. Culinary herbs are generally digestive aids, and although they may not be sufficiently estrogenic by themselves to reduce menopausal symptoms, they provide some help. Anything that improves digestion and absorption is likely to be beneficial to your well-being.

Hawthorn (*Crataegus species*)

Hawthorn has a long history as a heart and circulatory remedy. It helps blood flow by relaxing and strengthening the arteries. The main therapeutic compounds are various types of flavonoids, including procyanidins.[18]

It also has sedative, anti-inflammatory, and antioxidant effects. Usually, tablets or liquid extracts of the leaves, flowers, or berries are prescribed specifically for each patient, or a tea can be made from the berries.

Hawthorn can reduce flushing in postmenopausal women, and because it has sedative effects I recommend it for women who have nights sweats, insomnia, and palpitations. See a qualified practitioner, however, if you have a heart problem.

Saw Palmetto (*Serenoa repens*)

You're probably familiar with saw palmetto for its use in reducing urinary problems in men with benign prostatic hyperplasia (noncancerous swelling).[19]

Saw palmetto contains a relatively high level of phytosterols. One group of researchers reported that "the relatively high potency of beta-sitosterol is very marked compared with the other identified phytoestrogens."[20]

Historically, saw palmetto is an herb that has been surrounded by a number of contradictory myths in respect of breast enlarging, muscle building, and so on, none of which have any foundation. However, it does tend to lower testosterone activity in the body so it may be useful for women who have signs of high testosterone, such as facial hair growth and aggression.

I invariably include saw palmetto in a menopausal formula for women with irritable bladders, plus antiseptic herbs if an infection shows up in a urine test.

Chaste Tree (*Vitex agnus-castus*)

Chaste tree is, for me, a somewhat paradoxical herb. Traditionally, it was considered a female hormone balancer and an antilibido herb for men, which explains why it was formerly called "monk's pepper"! In herbal medicine, the berries are used to make tablets or extracts.

Chaste tree can affect prolactin, the hormone related to human breast milk, but in some circumstances (breast-feeding women) it has an increasing effect and in others (people with abnormally high prolactin) a decreasing effect. Of course, if you have abnormal breast secretions, you must consult a physician. A German study showed that chaste tree appeared to be more effective than vitamin B_6 for premenstrual syndrome (PMS).[21] It is helpful for acne and may help some cases of infertility. In Germany, doctors prescribe it for menstrual cycle irregularities, premenstrual complaints, and painful breasts.[22]

It is thought that chaste tree works via brain hormones and not directly on estrogen, progesterone, or testosterone, which is why it is difficult to be more precise.

I don't use chaste tree for menopausal symptoms unless women have acne, but many herbalists report it is effective and various manufacturers promote it for this purpose.

Are There Any Progesterogenic Plants?

The short answer to the question of whether there are any progesterogenic plants is, "Probably not." Although I was taught that there are plants that stimulate progesterone in the body, my subsequent search over twenty years has not revealed any clear evidence of any. Plants that were previously thought to have some type of progesterone activity—such as sarsaparilla, beth root, false unicorn, fenugreek, and wild yam—are more likely to be estrogenic if they are given at high medicinal doses. Given that progesterone and estrogen offset each other to some extent, the weaker phytoestrogens indirectly displace some of the body's strong estrogens in young women with high levels of estrogen. Progesterones may be more active in the body due to the possible antiestrogenic effect of some plant components, but that situation would not apply to menopausal women.

Many of the traditional hormonal herbs are helpful for menstrual problems, but because they may modify the pituitary and hypothalamus, their usefulness for menopausal and postmenopausal symptoms awaits further evaluation.

OTHER REMEDIES FOR MENOPAUSE
(AND GENERAL HEALTH)

Vitamin E

In August 1974, *Prevention* magazine circulated a questionnaire on menopause. There was no mention of vitamin E in the questionnaire, yet 2,000 women volunteered the information that this supplement had largely or totally relieved menopausal symptoms, including flushing and leg cramps, and improved well-being.

I recommend about 500 to 800 IU (335 to 537 milligrams) of vitamin E daily for this purpose, for three months, and then take a lower dose long term for your heart and circulation. You can also prick open a capsule to use as a face oil; if your skin is dry, you'll be surprised how quickly it is absorbed.

Other Vitamins

A number of the B vitamins enhance the action of estradiol although they have no estrogenic activity themselves. Taking a B-complex supplement may help menopausal stress, especially if combined with plant estrogens and vitamin C. Did you know that a severely stressed goat produces up to 100,000 milligrams of vitamin C a day? Humans don't make vitamin C in their bodies, but we're told that around 30 milligrams a day is adequate. I suggest about 3,000 mg a day, in divided doses, to help counteract stress.

Oils (for Internal Use)

Olive, linseed, corn, apricot kernel, wheat germ, and sesame oils are some of the recommended oils that can be included in the diet for their essential fatty acid content and to help maintain a healthy skin and vagina. Fish oil, evening primrose oil, and vitamin E are covered in more detail in chapters 9 and 10.

Oils for the Skin

Apricot kernel, sesame, and almond oils can also be used on the skin, but you may prefer to massage them into your skin thoroughly before shower-ing (unless your skin is very dry, in which case they can be applied after). You may also want to add a little aromatic lavender or rose oil to them, around ten to twenty drops to 3 ounces. As a face oil, you can also add a lit-tle sandalwood and basil oils, but you may need to tissue off the surplus before you go out.

Never put aromatic oils close to the eyes; it is very irritating. Be aware that some people are allergic to aromatic compounds.

St. John's Wort (*Hypericum perforatum*)

St. John's wort can be very helpful if you are feeling down, although it may cause a few side effects in sensitive people and may interact with some pharmaceuticals.

Kava (*Piper methysticum*)

If you are feeling anxious, try a course of kava.

Remedies That Don't Help Menopausal Symptoms

Dong Quai (*Angelica sinensis*)   An unbiased scientific trial of seventy-one women lasting twelve weeks showed that dong quai was not effective for relieving menopausal symptoms such as hot flashes and sweating.[23]

In traditional Chinese medicine, herbs are usually prescribed in formulas and based on an individual evaluation of each patient. This study does not mean that dong quai has no value, but when used singly in a European context it is apparently not effective for menopausal symptoms.

Evening Primrose Oil   Evening primrose oil suffers from overzealous promotion. Although it is promoted for menopausal symptoms in a number of countries, I could find no evidence or reason how it would work. One scientific trial confirmed that it offered no more benefit than placebo in treating menopausal flushing.[24]

Of course, evening primrose oil has various therapeutic benefits such as alleviating PMS and painful breasts, and I recommend it for all women on HRT.

Wild Yam Cream   Wild yam herb is a traditional colic remedy. The promotion of wild yam cream externally or a few drops under the tongue as a treatment for hormonal disorders, however, is based on misunderstanding and confusion and is so bizarre that I have covered it separately in appendix III.

General Recommendations for Menopause and Other Symptoms

For all symptoms, eat the foods and sprouts listed in chapters 3 and 4. Exercise is good for virtually everything and is covered in chapters 7 and 8. Relaxation, meditation, and pleasant social interaction are also beneficial and highly recommended for most problems.

Flushing   A selection of herbs for relieving flushing symptoms is given on pages 123 to 124. The ones most commonly prescribed are black cohosh and red clover.

Stress and Fatigue   Ginseng is commonly used to relieve stress and fatigue.

Insomnia   Hops is often recommended for insomnia.

If you're constantly rushing to "catch up" or if you don't have enough physical and mental activity, don't be surprised if you can't sleep well. Your body needs a balance of activity and rest, and regular lifestyle habits help promote restful sleep. Don't be one of those people who wake up feeling that you've worked all night!

Heart Palpitations   Hawthorn and motherwort herbs, and a medical checkup, are recommended for heart palpitations.

Vaginal Dryness   A number of women find that oils applied externally, such as vitamin E and almond oil, can relieve vaginal dryness, although they are somewhat messy to apply. Use only natural cold-pressed oils and avoid anything perfumed.

I've seen quite good results with licorice cream (see page 127), but whatever you use, always try a small test patch first because vaginal tissue is very sensitive.

Drugstores and health food stores often sell natural products. In some cases it may be necessary to use a natural estrogen cream, such as estriol.

Petroleum jelly is not cleared easily by the vagina and may promote infections. Water-based lubricants dry quickly after exposure to air.

Olive, fish, and evening primrose oils taken internally may help.

Menopausal Acne   Chaste tree can help relieve menopausal acne.

I have found the natural therapies given in this chapter to be helpful for relieving menopausal symptoms. Remember, though, that what you do to maintain your life in a state of relaxed alertness is usually more important than taking any remedy.

Suggestions for treating and preventing other problems related to heart, memory, and cancer are covered in chapter 9.

CHAPTER SIX

Osteoporosis and Bone Fractures

WHAT IS OSTEOPOROSIS?

The word *osteoporosis* means "porous bones." Each of the 206 bones in the human body is made up of a network of connective tissue fibers, and minerals are deposited within this framework. The connective tissue provides support, bone elasticity, and hardness, and the minerals fill the gaps to give strength. The mineral part of bones, technically called *apatite*, makes up about 65 percent of total bone weight; therefore, when you lose minerals from your bones, you lose quantity and strength. People with osteoporosis lose connective tissue through their urine, so osteoporosis is not just mineral loss.[1] Perhaps we should look more at on the quality of bone connective tissue rather than overemphasizing calcium and hormones.

Bones vary in shape and structure according to their function; for example, if you examine the leg of a cooked chicken (with the meat removed), you will see that the thickened ends are softer than the middle portion and that the outer layers are different from the inner segments. The outside part of bone is more compact (cortical), whereas the inside is a meshwork (trabecular), and both contribute to bone strength. Long bones such as the thigh are primarily cortical, whereas the uppermost thickened portion of the leg and the wrist are mainly trabecular.

Trabecular bone loss can begin as early as twenty years of age in both men and women. Cortical loss usually begins at about forty years, with women losing at about twice the rate of men. After menopause, some women go through a period of rapid trabecular loss for one or more years. Also, with aging, the compact portions may become "brittle" and the network portions may be too porous.

Bones are constantly changing. Stem cells give rise to osteoclasts (breakdown), which in turn gives rise to osteoblasts that produce new bone cells. In a growing child there is more osteoblast activity, in young adults it is about even, and in older people there is more breakdown activity. Various hormones are linked to bone strength and growth, including reproductive, adrenal, parathyroid, and growth hormones. In laboratory rats, a controlled deficiency of almost any hormone or nutrient will result in weakened bones. A number of enzymes and biochemical compounds are also related to bone strength. Genes, too, are linked to bone strength; black people, for example, don't have as much bone turnover as white people, which explains why they have stronger bones.[2]

A scan taken of one area of the body may not necessarily be indicative of the bone density in another area. Sometimes you can have good bone mineral levels (density) or bone mass (quantity) but still sustain a fracture.

WHAT CAUSES OSTEOPOROSIS?

Several factors may contribute to the development of osteoporosis, such as:

- Aging
- Poor nutrition
- Inadequate or excessive physical activity
- Sedentary lifestyle or periods of immobilization
- Excess bed rest (due to fatigue, illness, injury)
- Low calcium intake

- Excessive salt, sugar, or protein intakes
- Excess of a particular mineral
- Toxic metals
- Deficiency of any essential nutrient
- More than two alcoholic drinks per day
- Consuming two or more cups of coffee daily, especially black coffee
- Poor digestion
- Intestinal disorders such as Crohn's or celiac disease
- Cigarette smoking
- Fad dieting with weight loss and gain
- Some pharmaceuticals
- High acid-residue diet (e.g., excess meat)
- Digestive enzyme deficiencies
- Biochemical abnormalities
- Allergies/intolerances
- Excess phosphorus (as in soft drinks)
- Aspartame
- Depression
- Hypertension
- Adrenopause (male and female hormonal aging)
- Premature menopause
- Genes and family history of nontraumatic fractures
- Slight physical build and pale skin
- Eating disorders (past or current)
- Premenopausal history of amenorrhea (no periods)
- Multiple pregnancies
- Certain diseases, such as overactive thyroid
- Radiation therapy
- Inadequate sun exposure (or vitamin D deficiency)
- Fluoridated water

Some of these causes might produce only small, seemingly negligible effects, and any one of them may not be relevant, but a number of them over the long term are likely to affect bone health.

Although there is no certainty that these or any other risk factors could be used to predict either osteoporosis or fractures, they may provide a guide to prevention and be part of a treatment program. My experience is that patients are usually curious to know why they have a health problem. Often, however, there isn't a satisfactory explanation. In most cases, we don't know how long a person may have had osteoporosis because some surveys show that even a percentage of teenagers have low bone mineral density. In some cases, babies may be born with relatively weak bones, particularly if the mothers were on a poor diet during pregnancy.

The following sections provide brief explanations of some of these risk factors.

Hormonal Changes

The general agreement used to be that for up to five or ten years after menopause, many women have a marked increase in bone mineral loss and that this loss is greater in those who have had surgical or early menopause. Recent evidence indicates that "age-related changes become much more important, and half of the mass loss around the menopause is reversed without any intervention."[3]

One U.S. survey showed that 6 to 19 percent of people age twenty-five to thirty-four have abnormally low cortical bone density, and 22 percent of women age fifty-five to sixty-four lost little or no bone over an eleven-year period. My own clinical experience is that the greatest bone mineral loss occurs in the year after menstrual periods stop.

Insufficient Exercise

Based on personal experience and looking at over a hundred studies linking exercise to bone health, I am convinced that exercise is a major factor in building healthy bones. You've probably heard that once you're over fifty you can no longer improve your bones, muscle strength, and flexibility, but that is simply not true. I have seen marked improvements in my own classes.

During one menopause seminar I attended, an "expert" demonstrated exercises that involved sitting on a chair, straightening one leg, and pulling the toes back. Another exercise involved slowly moving the arms from side to side while sitting in a chair. This sort of exercise might be useful for a disabled ninety-year-old person who has suffered from multiple fractures from advanced osteoporosis, but this type of activity won't do anything to build your bones. On the other hand, you don't need to lift weights or run marathons either.

There is also some evidence that calcium supplementation helps bones when accompanied by exercise, and when you don't exercise, calcium absorption is reduced.[4] Boron, a trace element, also seems to be helpful only if accompanied by physical activity.

Nutritional Influences

Directly or indirectly, bones require *all* the forty-five essential nutrients, and these nutrients need to be taken in the appropriate quantities and effectively digested and absorbed.

- Megadosing on calcium or any single nutrient may cause imbalances of other nutrients. Iron absorption, for instance, is reduced by excess calcium.
- Vitamin D is essential for bone health and may be obtained from foods and sunlight exposure, but overdosing on this vitamin and its synthetic forms can produce adverse reactions.
- Experimentally, retinol (vitamin A) causes fractures in animals, and a Swedish study linked excess retinol to an increase in osteoporotic fractures in humans.[5] In Scandinavia a large portion of retinol intake comes from cod liver oil, so this supplement should be used with caution and only when a therapeutic need is shown. I suggest that if you eat fruit, vegetables, and fish, there is no need to take vitamin A supplements in any form. Natural beta-carotene would be a better choice if supplementation is required because the body converts it to vitamin A. Never exceed label dosages, particularly of vitamin A or vitamin D.

- Carbonated drinks (soft drinks) have been associated with an increased incidence of fractures.[6] Girls between thirteen and eighteen years of age consume an average of two cans of soft drinks a day; boys consume an average of three cans, and some people average more than five cans daily.

Dieting

At least 40 percent of the U.S. women diet to reduce weight, which causes detrimental changes in bones even if accompanied by exercising.[7]

I had one interesting case confirming this situation. A fifty-one-year-old woman came to me with mild osteoporosis. I prescribed a supplement, diet, and exercise program, which she said did not suit her. About a year later I met her in the street, and she looked terrible. When I asked how she was, she said that she had seen another naturopath, who prescribed a strict diet for her—mainly fruit and salads—plus walking, which had caused a dramatic weight loss. She said she felt great. I suggested that she have a bone mineral density scan. A few weeks later she came back to my clinic with her bone mineral density results. During that one year on her so-called health diet, she had gone from mild osteoporosis to severe, and the doctor informed her that she now had the bones of a ninety-year-old woman.

Many teenagers and young women are obsessed with being extremely slim. If they exercise excessively, restrict nutrition, or both, their periods may stop and minerals may be lost from their bones. Older people tend to lose interest in food and consume a monotonous diet, which does not provide ideal levels of all the essential nutrients. Pregnant women with inadequate diets give birth to infants with less bone mineral density than pregnant women with adequate diets. A few studies on teenage girls have shown that some already have weakened bones, proving that bones can deteriorate at any age.

Excess of Prolonged Bed Rest (Immobilization)

Periods of prolonged bed rest at any age can weaken the bones. In young people, moderate loss can be recouped with good nutrition and exercise, but it is much more difficult in older people. Habitually staying in bed for more than nine hours a day may be a factor in weakening bones, because even in normal sleep you lose more bone minerals than at other times of the day.

Digestion and Absorption Problems

Common sense says that even if you eat quality foods and supplements, you won't get the benefits if they are not absorbed into the body's cells. Your stomach contains acid and other compounds to break down food into absorbable particles; the liver and pancreas secrete bile and enzymes to aid absorption. Nutrients are absorbed mainly in the small intestines. Any areas or processes that are malfunctioning, inflamed, or irritated can lead to health problems, including osteoporosis.

Herbs that are bitter tasting, taken before meals, can aid digestion. Also, a little vinegar sprinkled on food might improve digestion; a study on laboratory rats showed that vinegar improved calcium solubility and prevented osteoporosis.[8]

HERBAL VINEGAR

2 teaspoons turmeric powder
2 teaspoons ginger powder
1 to 2 teaspoons crushed caraway seeds
½ teaspoon hot chili powder
  Contents of 2 chamomile teabags
  Large handful of chopped fresh herbs (such as peppermint, oregano, tarragon, basil)
1 pint apple cider vinegar

Put the ingredients into a bottle. Seal, label, and date the bottle and store it on its side for at least a few days before use.

The vinegar acts as a preservative and draws out the components of the herbs. The herbs increase the digestive action of the vinegar. (Any dried or fresh culinary herbs can be used for this purpose.)

Sprinkle 2 teaspoons on salads or savory meals or use in a salad dressing. (More is not better; you don't want too much extra acid in your stomach!)

Foods and herbs containing inulin and fructooligosaccharides (the nondigestible carbohydrates found in fruits, vegetables, and other plants) help by acting as building blocks for the beneficial bacteria in your intestines, where absorption takes place. If you don't have the right bacterial balance, your digestion and elimination are impaired. Scientific researchers are suggesting that these types of compounds may indirectly improve the body's absorption of calcium and help with lipid metabolism.[9]

Some recommended herbs for improving digestion and increasing beneficial bacteria are the following:

- Aloes
- Burdock
- Chicory
- Dandelion
- Ginger
- Gotu kola
- Hot chili (small quantities)
- Licorice
- Milk thistle
- Slippery elm
- All culinary herbs

Some recommended foods and supplements for improving digestion are the following:

- Whey powder
- Shiitake mushrooms
- Fish oil
- Evening primrose oil
- Fruits and vegetables
- Soluble fiber such as psyllium
- Tofu
- Chlorella and seaweeds
- Rice bran
- Antioxidants, especially beta-carotene and vitamin C

Calcium metabolism is significantly stimulated by fructooligosaccharides. Studies with rats suggest that fructooligosaccharides may increase calcium absorption by 30 percent in the intestines.[10] Fructooligosaccharides are also available as supplements.

Avoid foods and drinks that upset your digestive system or cause allergy or sensitivity reactions, such as lactose intolerance. In Australia it is estimated that 19 percent of whites between ages nineteen and sixty-one are lactose intolerant, which means that they do not have the enzyme required to digest the sugar in milk. A New Zealand study of elderly women with an average age of sixty-six showed that 61 percent were lactose intolerant.[11] The signs of this absorption problem include abdominal bloating and cramps, flatulence, and diarrhea. In fact, milk might be making some people's bones worse because anything that causes digestive problems means that the digestive system is irritated and consequently doesn't absorb nutrients efficiently. If your bowel movements are watery, nutrients are passing through the intestines too quickly and many nutrients will be excreted rather than be absorbed. Hence, laxatives should be used with caution.

Pharmaceutical Drugs

A number of pharmaceuticals—notably anti-inflammatory cortisone drugs (glucocorticoids), some diuretics, some laxatives, anticoagulants such as heparin, analgesics, antacids, anticonvulsants, thyroid medications, calcium antagonists, and some weight-reducing drugs—can weaken bones. Indirectly, some of the new cholesterol-lowering drugs and so-called smart fats that reduce blood cholesterol may reduce bone strength because they not only mop up cholesterol but also other fat-soluble nutrients necessary for bone and nutrient metabolism. You don't want your cholesterol to get too low because cholesterol has many functions in the body, including hormone metabolism, and hormones are also associated with bone metabolism.

Toxic Metals

Aluminum   Aluminum can accumulate in bones, and it decreases bone-building activity. Avoid cooking with aluminum cookware because aluminum can upset the parathyroid gland, which in turn affects your bones. Also, some antacids contain aluminum.

Cadmium, Lead, and Other Toxic Compounds   Long-term exposure of cadmium causes softening of the bones. Toxic metals such as cadmium and lead are hard to avoid because they are in our food and environment and get stored in our bones. Be aware, however, that if you diet excessively, these toxic metals come out of the bones and circulate in the blood, potentially causing depression, anxiety, and memory problems. I buy and grow some organic foods to reduce cadmium and pesticide exposure.

Iron   Iron overload can cause a number of problems, including reducing the absorption of calcium and other minerals. Unless you have medically diagnosed iron deficiency anemia, you don't need to take iron supplements.

Cigarette Smoking

At least thirteen studies link smoking to osteoporosis.[12] Cigarette smoking is a major risk factor for fractures and is associated with increased free radical levels and decreased antioxidant levels. Current smokers with low intakes of both vitamin E and vitamin C had a 4.9-fold higher risk of hip fractures, according to one survey.[13]

It has also been demonstrated that smokers' bones heal more slowly than nonsmokers' bones. Women who smoke twenty cigarettes each day throughout their adult lives will have a 5 to 10 percent deficit in bone density at menopause. Smoking is also linked to wrinkles as well as depression and anxiety symptoms.[14]

Excess Acid Residue From the Diet

When the body is loaded with acids, it responds by releasing alkaline compounds, such as calcium stored in bones, to buffer the excess acid in the body. In a typical Western diet that is relatively high in protein, a small amount of acid is generated daily; to offset this acid, calcium is pulled out of the bones. When potassium bicarbonate was given to postmenopausal women, it neutralized acid production from protein.[15] Vegetables are the most common food source of potassium, so always include them in a meal with a meat.

The findings of the 1997 Symposium of the Nutrition Working Group of the American Society for Bone and Mineral Research, Cincinnati, showed that a typical American diet that is high in protein and low in vegetables and fruits relates to bone loss and that increased intake of vegetables, fruit, and milk may compensate for the adverse effects that can result from a diet rich in meat.[16] These findings do not mean that a protein-deficient diet is good for the bones, and some types of vegetarians may be somewhat low in protein, which can lead to weakened bones.[17]

Swiss researchers have summarized the protein question very well by suggesting that vegans on a low-calorie diet might well benefit from increased protein intake. Someone having lunch at McDonald's every day, on the other hand, might be better off restricting [animal] protein intake.[18]

Depression

There is a link between depression and osteoporosis, possibly because when you are depressed, you tend not to exercise and or eat properly.

Hypertension

High blood pressure is associated with abnormalities in calcium metabolism, and a study of 3,700 elderly women confirmed that hypertension increases the risk of osteoporosis.[19]

Aspartame

A short-term study using aspartame (Nutrasweet) showed that it increases urinary calcium. The researchers recommended that until long-term studies prove otherwise, people with a history of kidney stones or weak bones should avoid aspartame.[20] Soft drinks feature prominently on the top twenty items purchased in supermarkets. Many of these drinks not only contain aspartame but are also high in phosphorus, which is also potentially harmful for bones.[21] In addition, a high sugar intake increases calcium excretion in the urine.

DO YOU HAVE OSTEOPOROSIS?

Signs and Risk Factors

Your bones may be osteoporotic if you fracture a bone as a result of a very minor fall or during your normal daily activities.

Not everyone with poor posture has osteoporosis. Sometimes people are born with curvatures or they habitually stoop or slump. I have seen a number of frail, elderly patients with excellent carriage but who have severe osteoporosis. I have also seen many young people whose bones are strong but who have the posture of an eighty-year-old osteoporotic.

Some outward signs of weakening bones may be a dowager's hump, loss of height, thin body, weak muscles, poor muscle definition, periodontal disease (wasting gums or tooth loss), premature gray hair, premature wrinkles, and thin skin. (Back pain is not generally linked to osteoporosis except in extreme cases.)

A medical diagnosis is the only reasonably accurate way of knowing the state of your bone health.

Medical Diagnosis

Various biochemical tests of urine and blood may be indicators of bone health, but at the moment, osteoporosis and fracture risk are assessed by

- Single- or dual-energy X-ray absorptiometry (scan)
- Quantitative computed tomography (scan)
- Ultrasound (relatively new)

It is beyond the scope of this chapter to explain the technical details of these diagnostic tools, but in general, an X-ray scan gives less radiation and is less expensive than quantitative computed tomography. Ultrasound is not fully tested, and the opinion of most practitioners is that testing the heel may not be a reliable means of assessing what is happening in your hip (upper femur) and lower spine, which are the crucial fracture areas of an aging body.

These measuring techniques are not perfect. For example, an X-ray scan may not always be accurate in obese people or in those with arthritic calcification. Also, there are variations in equipment and techniques, so any subsequent tests should be done with the same equipment at the same center. Your physician will be aware of these variations. Test results often indicate a percentage in relation to healthy young women and to healthy women in your age group so you can see how you compare. It is desirable to be at least close to the levels found in healthy women in your age group or more than 85 percent of the levels in healthy young women. The report may, however, summarize your situation scientifically in terms of standard deviations (comparative risk). For example:

Fifty-one-year-old woman with an L2–L4 (lower spine) reading of 0.759 g/cm²

This reading is 2.73 standard deviations below the average for a young
    normal woman (the T score).
More than 2.50 standard deviations below equals significant mineral loss
    or osteoporosis.
Between 1.5 and 2.5 standard deviations below means osteopenia (weakness).
Between 0 and 1.5 standard deviations below is considered normal.

In simpler language, a lower spine (L2–L4) actual reading should be 1.00 g/cm² or more and the femoral neck (upper leg) reading should be above 85 g/cm² for a fifty- to fifty-five-year-old. (This standard varies somewhat between countries.)

If this explanation is too complicated for you, ask your health practitioner for a simpler explanation in terms of comparing your bones with those of healthy women in your age group.

Unfortunately, there may be variations or errors in the calculations. If your report does not make sense after you have studied this segment, your scan results, and the accompanying scan report, ask your physician for an explanation.

Osteoporotic Fracture

A fracture that occurs during normal daily activities or from minor mishaps is called an *osteoporotic fracture*. A bone broken by a serious fall or accident is called a *traumatic fracture*. When fractures occur in elderly people, it is commonly a hip fracture, that is the hip in the narrow part of the upper leg (the neck of the femur) that fractures, simply because it is the narrowest part. Occasionally, other parts of the upper leg and hip joint are involved in osteoporotic fractures. In very frail elderly people, a crush fracture (collapse) can occur in the lower spine. These types of fractures are very rare in people under the age of fifty. Women with weak wrists and inflexible feet—a trend I have noticed in my yoga classes—are more likely to have fractures in these areas.

WHAT CAUSES FRACTURES?

Osteoporosis is the major cause of fractures in women over fifty, and many of these fractures are classed as nontraumatic, that is, breaking a bone in the foot from tripping on a step or crushing a spinal vertebra when getting out of a chair. Some studies, however, show that almost half the fractures suffered by women over fifty actually occur in those designated as having normal bones, so there are obviously causes other than low bone mineral density. I have seen patients who have sustained fractures from relatively minor falls with slow recovery periods, yet their bones were excellent according to bone mineral density scans.

Studies in the United States and Italy have shown a link between coffee intake and hip fractures.[22] In Italy the link between milk and cheese consumption was found to be very weak.[23] Again, these studies point to the overemphasis of milk and dairy foods as a means of preventing fractures.

Furthermore, bone density scans do not reveal the state of the bone collagen, which may partially explain why some osteoporotic women have quite serious accidents yet do not sustain fractures. More studies need to examine this category of women with low bone mineral density who don't suffer fractures.

One woman I saw who had extremely severe osteoporosis was hit by a car with such force that she was thrown over the hood but, amazingly, sustained only one small fracture in her foot plus cuts and bruising. Meanwhile, a yoga student of mine, a solidly built, very fit woman with a bone density reading that was better than the average healthy young woman, sustained a serious leg fracture from a minor fall down one step, and it took many months to heal.

The message is *not* to avoid exercise because your bones are weak, but I am not recommending high-impact aerobics or skydiving either.

Reduced Muscle and Joint Strength

Muscles and joints also provide strength and protect the bones. If you don't use your muscles and joints, they become weaker and less flexible. There also needs to be a degree of flexibility in the joints (and bones) to provide a "cushioning" effect, especially from accidents. Many women who come to my clinic have poor posture and look ten years older than their biological age, not because they have osteoporosis but because they have not adequately exercised their muscles and joints and have a lifelong habit of poor posture.

Falls

About 90 percent of hip fractures result from falls, so maintaining your physical fitness will avoid, reduce, or absorb the force of any fall. Causes of falls include the following:

- Lack of postural control, weak muscles, and diminished reflexes.
- Unstable joints. (As you age, your joint structures tend to wear away. Doing only one type of exercise might lead to your joints "wearing" unevenly, and this instability could cause more falls and fractures. A variety of physical activity is recommended.)
- Feet and walking problems. (Your feet are the foundation of your entire body, and the way you stand and walk affects your knees, hips, and spine. Looking after your feet is good advice for everyone.)

- Inappropriate shoes.
- Poor eyesight.
- Dizziness and ear problems.
- Confusion or dementia.
- Insomnia (insufficient sleep can make you careless).
- Impatience (accidents often occur when you are rushing or not concentrating).
- Diseases such as arthritis, Parkinson's disease, circulatory and heart problems, or multiple sclerosis.
- Alcoholism.
- Pharmaceutical drugs, including sedatives and some hypertension medications.
- Poor lighting.
- Environmental hazards such as electricity cords and floor rugs. (Use nonslip mats, don't leave things lying on the floor, don't place furniture and other obstacles near entries, paint the edges of outdoor steps a light color, and have a rounded finish on concrete surfaces in the yard.)

Be sensible without being timid or reckless. Older people are sometimes advised to restrict their physical activities, not to walk on uneven surfaces, and so on, but if you listened to all this advice you could end up housebound and immobile.

Fluoride

Bone fluorosis means that the structure of the bones is altered in such a way that fractures are more likely to occur. In parts of India, the excessive fluoride content of soil, water, and food causes mottling of teeth, bone problems, low hemoglobin, and thyroid problems. Other studies show that fluoride is toxic to the nervous system.[24]

It is now known that fluoride accumulates with age and may reach toxic levels in bone during a person's lifetime if the water supply is fluoridated. In the United States a number of studies have shown an increased inci-

dence of osteoporosis and hip fracture with even low-dose water fluoridation. One researcher has stated that fluoridation is unsafe.[25] Thus, total
daily fluoride exposure should be reduced, the contaminant fluoride level
should be lowered, and the addition of fluoride to public drinking water
should be ended.

WHO GETS OSTEOPOROTIC FRACTURES?

Bone fractures in older men and women are increasing rapidly, likely due to
decreasing physical activity, modern diets, and lifestyle habits. Table 6.1
illustrates the relationship of hip fractures to diet. People are also living
longer. Hip fractures are commonly linked to osteoporosis and old age, but
not all elderly people get osteoporotic fractures.

In one study of elderly women, only eighteen of sixty-one hip fractures
occurred in the so-called high-risk group.[26]

TABLE 6.1 **Relationship Between Intake of Animal
Protein and Calcium to Hip-Fracture Rate**

	Hip Fracture Rate per 100,000 People	Animal Protein Intake (g/day)	Calcium Intake (mg/day)
Norway	190.4	66.6	1,087
United States	144.9	72.0	973
New Zealand	119.0	77.8	1,217
Yugoslavia	27.6	27.3	588
Hong Kong	45.6	34.6	356
Singapore	21.6	24.7	389
South Africa (blacks)	6.8	10.4	196

Source: M. Messina and V. Messina, *The Simple Soybean and Your Health* (New York: Avery, 1994), p. 114.

It has been shown that daughters of osteoporotic women are not more prone to sustain fractures than the rest of the population, so don't believe that a fracture is inevitable. Remember that you can inherit diet and lifestyle habits that can cause weak bones.

A number of studies have shown that people on a low-calcium diet may actually adapt and be able to attain high levels of calcium absorption.

Sedentary Lifestyles and Fractures

A Swedish survey suggests that fractures of the hip are increasing in elderly men.[27] The Australian Bureau of Statistics' figures for men indicate that about 21 percent more men than women die as a result of a fractured femur. This finding suggests that perhaps elderly women are more durable than elderly men.

Although osteoporosis causes a considerable burden on health resources, many media reports and some scientific papers give exaggerated figures about the number of people who die as a result of osteoporotic fractures. Table 6.2 gives the number of deaths relating to fractures for women in Australia.

The total number of deaths from neck of femur (hip) fractures, 314, are probably all osteoporosis related, and this figure is included in the total of 461.

A study in regional Australia showed that fracture incidence rates were higher in women (29.5 per 1,000 person-years) than men (14.4 per 1,000 person-years). All fracture patients had a higher risk of death in the first year after a fracture, particularly in the over sixty-nine age group, with about one-third more men dying compared with women.[28]

There are many interesting differences between various countries. For example:

- Greek women have about 50 percent fewer fractures than women in the United States. A dietary and lifestyle survey suggested that the consumption of olive oil (which is rich in vitamin E) in conjunction with other lifestyle factors may be an explanation.[29] Perhaps

TABLE 6.2 **Number of Female Deaths Relating to Fractures in 1998**

Age Group	Fracture, Cause Unspecified	Fracture, Where Neck of Femur (hip) Was Listed in the Death Certificates
20–24	1	0
55–59	1	0
60–64	2	2
65–69	5	3
70–74	9	7
75–79	46	29
80–84	79	55
85 +	318	218
All ages	461	314

Source: Australian Bureau of Statistics.

Notes: Some of these fractures may have been caused by accidents.

The United States has a population about fifteen times greater than Australia, so the figures are likely to be that much higher in the United States.

Greek women get more sunlight (vitamin D) and are not as weight-obsessed as women in the United States.

- American and Norwegian men have a higher hip fracture rate than English women.
- In the former Yugoslavia there was not a great deal of difference between male and female fracture rates.
- Swedish women have seventeen times the fracture rate of Polish women.
- Bantu men have a slightly higher fracture rate than Bantu women.
- Japanese women are generally of small stature and have low calcium intakes, but they have a low rate of hip and other fractures compared with European women.

- In developed, industrialized countries such as the United States, a low calcium intake is consistently linked to fracture risk, yet the Bantus of South Africa have the lowest calcium intakes in the world but the lowest age-matched fracture incidence.

Medical Options for Treating Osteoporosis

Hormone Replacement Therapy   Hormone replacement therapy generally helps prevent bone loss and sometimes gives a small increase in bone mineral density. As discussed in chapter 2 and appendix I, HRT carries a long list of potential adverse effects and needs to be taken continuously for the benefit to be sustained. If you take HRT for five years after menopause, the bone loss accelerates when the hormones are stopped. The bone mineral density of women who have stopped HRT after ten years is similar to that in women who have never taken menopausal hormones.[30]

A number of researchers report that HRT may have little residual effect on bone density among women seventy-five years of age and older, who have the highest risk of fracture.[31]

Androgen Therapy   Testosterone is sometimes prescribed in conjunction with estrogen. Men have bigger bones and muscles than women because they have a higher level of androgens (male hormones).

Nandrolone and related compounds can have masculinizing effects in women. These androgen medications are usually prescribed when HRT is not advisable.

Even though some researchers suggest that androgen deficiency may be of greater importance than estrogen deficiency in postmenopausal bone loss, women are unlikely to become enthusiastic about using these types of hormones.

Parathyroid, DHEA, and Other Hormones   Parathyroid, DHEA, and other hormones may be effective in some cases, but all hormone therapies need to be prescribed with care according to individual requirements.

Alendronate   Alendronate is a bisphosphonate recommended for treating postmenopausal osteoporosis. It can have gastrointestinal side effects, which could reduce absorption over the long term. A number of different types of bisphosphonates are now available for prescription. The concern is that overtreatment could suppress bone remodeling completely and thus impair the ability of the skeleton to repair microfractures and other structural damage.[32]

Etidronate   I have seen a few patients who experienced dramatic bone mineral losses while taking the pharmaceutical etidronate, as well as some with severe skin rashes and other adverse reactions.

Raloxifene   Raloxifene is a selective estrogen receptor modulator (SERM), which is less effective than HRT on bones but is not linked to breast cancer risk. It may increase blood clotting diseases.

Alendronate and raloxifene were both recently approved for the prevention of postmenopausal osteoporosis, although their efficacy has not been fully evaluated.[33] Women at low risk for hip fracture, heart disease, and breast cancer do not benefit significantly from any such treatment.

Calcitonin   Calcitonin is derived from salmon and is much stronger than human calcitonin. In some countries it is available as an injection or can be deposited into the nose.

Fluoride   Fluoride increases bone mineral density by about 10 percent per year, but that does not reflect an increase in bone strength.[34] One-third of patients treated with fluoride experience gastric irritation, and one-third have leg pain. Because there is no decrease in fracture rates, it does not seem a worthwhile therapy.

Thiazide Diuretics   Thiazide diuretics reduce bone loss, but their effects on fracture incidence have not been determined. Because diuretics can increase mineral excretion, the long-term effects on fracture in the elderly remain questionable.

Natural Progesterone   Although natural progesterone, notably in the form of a skin cream, has been promoted as a bone builder, its proponents have used it in conjunction with nutritional supplements, diet, lifestyle adjustments, and sometimes estrogen. A scientifically controlled study has now been completed in Pennsylvania on 102 women, and after one year there was no significant difference between the bone mineral density of the women on the progesterone cream and those on the placebo. Both groups were also prescribed a multivitamin and a calcium, and both had similar, slight reductions in bone mineral density.[35]

Although the promoters of natural progesterone cream suggest that the bone results are better with older women, that has not been scientifically evaluated. In the Pennsylvania trial, however, natural progesterone cream improved or resolved 83 percent of those experiencing hot flashes, compared with 19 percent of those on the placebo cream.

Ipriflavone   Ipriflavone is a synthetic flavonoid that prevents bone loss in osteoporotic women.[36] This medication is well tolerated, according to more than sixty studies done to date, and long-term use is considered safe. At least one researcher has suggested using ipriflavone together with a comprehensive bone-building vitamin and mineral program.[37]

In cases of established osteoporosis, it would seem advisable to combine ipriflavone with some nutrient supplementation plus an appropriate exercise program.

Calcitriol   Calcitriol is a vitamin D metabolite that is much more powerful than the over-the-counter vitamin D supplement. It has a long list of side effects and interactions with other drugs and nutrients.

Combination Therapies   Various combinations have been tested. One such combination is estrogen injections, cyclical etidronate, and 1 gram of calcium daily. After four years, this therapy increased the vertebrae bone mineral density by 10.9 percent and the femoral neck by 7.25 percent.[38]

Implants of estrogen and testosterone were more effective in increasing bone mineral density in the hip and spine than estradiol implants alone.[39]

If you go on any of these pharmaceuticals, you need to discuss all the risks and benefits with your doctor so that an individual assessment can be made to find the most appropriate treatment for you. Exercise along with good nutrition are just as important if you are taking pharmaceuticals, but you will need to discuss supplements with your doctor. For instance, if you are prescribed calcitriol, a metabolite of vitamin D, you should not take calcium or an additional vitamin D tablet.

Duration of Treatment

The general consensus is that a one- or two-year program is the most appropriate time for evaluating osteoporosis, because change does not occur quickly. A shorter time may not be valid because of adaptation; that is, the body gets to a certain level after a few months, and then further effects are weaker or zero.

None of these drugs is guaranteed to prevent fractures. There's also no guarantee that good nutrition and daily exercise will prevent fractures either, but they will improve your chances of living to a healthy old age.

CHAPTER SEVEN

Exercise: Your Bones' Best Friend

*T*he purpose of this chapter is to convince you that exercise will improve your bones—and just about everything else. Sedentary habits put you at risk for illness and early death from several diseases.

It is reasonable to assume that normal walking will not do much to strengthen your arms, nor will push-ups do much to strengthen your hips. You have 206 bones and 285 skeletal muscles in your body, and they all benefit from activity. Try to do a variety of physical activities and bring exercise into your daily life as much as possible. For instance:

- Walk up stairs instead of using escalators or elevators.
- If you work all day, delegate some semisedentary domestic chores such as ironing so that you have time and energy for more vigorous activities such as cleaning the car or going to the gym. Gardening and mowing the lawn are better for your bones than sewing, cooking, and washing dishes. Let other household members take on some of the repetitive light chores, which make you tired but have no health benefits.
- Do abdominal and gluteal squeezes while you are washing the dishes or talking on the phone.

- Bend your knees while vacuuming, keeping your back straight.
- Squat for some of the time while gardening; it strengthens the hip joint.
- Whenever practical, walk instead of using your car or public transportation.
- If you're looking after children, take them to a park and play physical games with them.
- When you're at home, dress in clothes that allow you to exercise or dance in case the mood hits you.
- Incorporate more physical activity into your day, watch less television, and avoid your computer!

Vitamin E and ginseng may help you exercise more effectively, particularly when you're getting started on your new program. If you eat plenty of vegetables and fruit (at least 5 cups a day), you don't need to take antioxidant supplements. The oxidative stress resulting from strenuous or exhaustive exercise is prevented, however, if 1,200 IU vitamin E (800 milligrams) supplementation is taken 12 and 2 hours before and 22 hours after.[1] Unless you're a long-distance runner, one dose a day of both ginseng and vitamin E is sufficient, and they should be taken in the morning. A reasonable dosage of vitamin E is about 600 IU (400 milligrams) a day.

STOP MAKING EXCUSES FOR NOT EXERCISING

Is Exercising Natural?

Exercising is probably not natural. It's obvious that most people don't like to exercise. When we have sufficient food and shelter, there is a natural inclination to loll around.

Adult hunter-gatherers apparently did not engage in sports or running except as part of gathering food. Experts estimate that stone-age adults would have typically spent about fifteen hours a week collecting food and would have engaged in other physical activity, such as making tools, collecting wood, and (probably) fighting. In other words, they had about twenty hours a week of low to moderate activity, with a small proportion of strenuous activity such as climbing trees and chasing animals.

Compare this lifestyle with that of a person who drives to work, sits down most of the day in front of a computer, watches television at night, and may have occasional bouts of strenuous activity such as a game of racquetball. It's no wonder we are weak and stressed.

Mental Barriers to Overcome

"I'm Healthy Enough" One of my patients had the "I'm healthy enough" attitude, but after I managed to persuade her to have a full fitness assessment at a medical sports center, she was shocked to learn that her level of fitness was the equivalent of a seventy-year-old. (She was twenty-five and is now improving her diet and lifestyle.)

"I'm Looking for Something I Enjoy" Some people think that they'll exercise when they find something they like, but after fifty years or so they still haven't found anything that appeals to them. Think of exercise as part of your job or as insurance. At the very least, buy some walking shoes and start walking.

"My Feet Hurt" The feet hurting excuse has about twenty variations, including "I hurt my knee in an accident." Get help for the problem. Most people can swim without pain (and if you don't know how to swim, take lessons). Any exercise helps, although some activities build bones better than others. Swimmers, for example, have strong arm bones. An exercise bike is another option.

"I'm Too Tired" Why are you so tired? Are you getting enough sleep? Are you anemic? Do you have an undiagnosed illness? Do you need to reorganize your time and lifestyle? If you can't identify the reason for your fatigue, you may need the help of a practitioner.

"I'm Too Busy" If you can't spare thirty minutes a day to exercise, you are doing too much. Many of our health problems are related to the stress of trying to do too much and trying to acquire too many things. In Ayurvedic medicine it is called the "loss of knowingness"; that is, we've lost the ability of knowing what is important and good.

"Exercise Makes Me Uncomfortable"   If you're not used to being puffed and sweaty, you may have some anxiety initially. If you don't feel anything, you haven't exercised, but you should not feel pain.

"I Don't Have Any Willpower"   Take a look at yourself in a full-length mirror. What has your lack of willpower done to your body?

Organize a small walking group; if you're the leader you have to show up. Combine some activity with pleasure; for example, plan weekend outings such as a long walk along the beach before lunch (preferably, with cheerful companions). Go on a vacation where you will be physically active.

"My Neighbor Was a Jogger Who Had a Heart Attack and Died on the Side of the Road"   Other variations on this theme include "Aunt Bessie didn't do any more than walk to the kitchen and she lived until she was ninety-seven." These examples are exceptions and probably relate to good or bad luck, hereditary characteristics, and so on.

"I've Never Exercised, and It's Too Late to Begin Now"   Nursing home residents in their nineties had an average increase of 4.2 percent in bone mineral density of the forearm after performing mild exercises for thirty minutes three times weekly for three years.[2] Those in the nursing home who didn't do the exercise program lost 2.5 percent of their bone mineral density.

Women ages fifty to seventy-three who exercised for one hour twice a week over eight months showed a 3.5 percent increase in lumbar spine bone mineral density. A number of other studies showed similar results. One of my patients who had a habitual sedentary lifestyle and didn't want to take any pills gained 8 percent in the bone mineral density of her femoral neck (upper leg/hip) after one year of a program designed for her at a fitness center. She did the program four times weekly for one hour, although at the beginning the activities were very light.

The time for excuses is over. There is no certainty that another time in the future will be more convenient than now.

EXERCISE IMPROVES BONE AND MUSCLE STRENGTH

Nearly every survey confirms that physically fit women, both menstruating and menopausal, have higher bone density than sedentary women. The exceptions are those who excessively exercise and who are fanatical about being extremely thin or extremely fit. Here are just a few examples of studies that confirm the benefits of physical activity.

- In ranked female tennis players, the bone of the playing arm is 28 percent thicker than that of the nonplaying arm.
- At middle age, the lumbar vertebrae of lifelong runners are 30 percent higher density than that of nonathletic women.[3] Older athletic women can have the same bone density as younger athletic women.
- In sedentary postmenopausal women, bone mineral content of lumbar vertebrae improved by 5.2 percent after nine months of exercises at 70 to 90 percent of maximal oxygen uptake for fifty to sixty minutes three times a week, whereas the control, nonexercising group lost 1.4 percent of their bone mass.[4]
- You don't have to be a superb athlete to get benefits. A one-year study of healthy, sedentary, early postmenopausal women showed that there was not much difference between a high-impact and low-impact exercise program of one hour a week.[5]
- When women between age sixty to ninety-eight were studied, those who reported long-term moderate exercise had better immune function based on blood tests compared with sedentary women.[6]
- Postmenopausal women who walked for thirty minutes a day for three to four days a week, after three weeks were asked to increase their walking speed and maintain it for forty to forty-five minutes daily. Not only were their fitness levels better, but their blood pressure readings were significantly decreased over the twelve weeks of exercise training.[7]

- In a study of 17,321 men, vigorous exercise, as compared with sedentary lifestyle, was related to a longer life.[8] The same would apply to women. Vigorous exercise included brisk walking, swimming laps, and playing tennis.
- Exercise may positively influence mood and anxiety.[9] It has also been shown that anxiety and depression are alleviated when people look at trees and water as opposed to traffic and buildings, so aim to get some of your activity in a natural surrounding.
- A high-fiber diet together with physical activity may also prevent diverticular disease.[10]
- Regular aerobic exercise has also been linked with a lowered incidence of gallstones.[11] One study showed that intraocular pressure reduced by 20 percent after three months of aerobic training.[12] Another showed that regular exercise increased DHEAs.[13] This hormone is being promoted as an antiaging product, but isn't it wiser to get more of this hormone from a healthy activity than from a pill? And, it's free.

One to two hours a week of walking or cycling can improve bone density. If you are already exercising for more than two hours a week, adding more of the same sort of exercise is unlikely to increase bone density, and you may have to look at other causes for your weak bones. (Chapter 6 lists possible causes of osteoporosis.)

With regular exercise, your joints and muscles become both stronger and more flexible. Physical activity is the only way to build muscles. Some thin people actually have low muscle content compared with body fat and are at a greater risk of osteoporotic fractures than heavier people.

The Benefits of Exercise

Appropriate exercise will help you live longer and healthier. It specifically improves:

- Bone and muscle strength and elasticity
- Heart and circulation

- Breathing and oxygen-carrying capacity
- Metabolic rate (you burn up more calories and have a leaner body)
- Joint tissue
- Blood fats and glucose levels
- Sleep
- Immune functioning
- Skin quality and general appearance
- Hormone balance
- Energy
- Emotional well-being
- Confidence and self-esteem
- Elimination of body wastes (via sweat, lymphatic system, urinary system, and feces)
- Physical appearance
- Reflexes and coordination
- Life span

Fitness and Independence   A U.S. report found that 40 percent of women between ages fifty-five and sixty-four, 45 percent between ages sixty-five and seventy-four, and 65 percent between ages seventy-five and eighty-four could not lift 10 pounds (4.5 kilograms).[14] This finding is alarming because it demonstrates muscle weakness in relatively young women. Weak muscles are a cause of falls, reduced mobility, and disability. Worst of all, 46 percent of American women between ages sixty-five and sixty-nine will be dependent on others during their remaining years. Enough studies have been done to show that even very old and frail people can increase strength and activity. If you want to remain mobile and independent, you must have regular physical activity.

Which Is the Best Exercise to Improve Bone Strength?

Weight-bearing exercise is the best way to improve bone strength. Such exercise includes walking, jogging, and dancing. Studies confirm, however, that walking and dancing do not increase bone mineral density in the arms. Rowing may be more effective than brisk walking in promoting spinal bone growth.

Light aerobic activity, usually thirty to fifty minutes three to four times weekly, has shown the best results. Programs using light weights are also successful. Lifting weights may also be more strengthening for spinal bone than walking is. Weight training leads to significant gains in muscle strength, size, and functional mobility among frail residents of nursing homes up to ninety-six years of age.[15]

At least fifteen studies have shown that elderly people can improve their strength and endurance through weight training. Excessive repetitive weight work or doing only one type of exercise, however, can markedly aggravate arthritis. Initially, you need supervision rather than encouragement from younger enthusiastic bodybuilders. If you are unaccustomed to intense physical exercise, a rigorous program late in life may actually cause more falls or place too much force on bones and joints that are not adapted to such high stresses.[16]

Exercising your upper legs with leg toners or weights is more likely to improve the upper leg and hip bones and allow you to walk longer distances. If you can't walk, you lose your independence.

An overall program suitable for older people is a combination of walking briskly (or some similar activity) for thirty minutes three times weekly and for another thirty minutes three times weekly doing a variety of strengthening, mobilizing, and balance exercises similar to the ones outlined below or under supervision at a fitness center.

Circuit training is also excellent if you like the fitness center atmosphere. In circuit training you spend a few minutes on various types of equipment such as rowing machines, bikes, arm strengtheners, and leg toners, as well as doing some floor exercises. Centers may have more than twenty different types of equipment.

The simple fact is that if you want a healthy body, you have to be active.

Overexercising

A number of young athletes and ballet dancers sustain injuries and damage from overexercising and undereating. In over twenty years of clinical practice, I have seen few women over fifty who overexercise, although many work too hard.

A two-year study compared twenty-seven exercisers and thirteen nonexercisers over fifty. In both males and females, measurement of the lumbar spine showed that exercising at moderate levels was beneficial to bone mineral density. An interesting finding was that excessive exercise apparently causes low spinal bone densities compared with levels in those exercising less vigorously. In this study, excessive exercise for females over fifty was defined as jogging for more than 300 minutes a week.[17]

What If You Already Have Osteoporosis?

If you already have osteoporosis, caution should be observed, particularly in the early stages of a new exercise program. That doesn't mean resigning yourself to boring, low-stress introductory classes, although they may be a starting point.

Shorter periods of varied, light activities are advised. If you join a class, always tell the teacher about any health problems you may have.

Swimming is an excellent exercise, and although you may have heard that it does not improve bones, studies have shown that swimmers have stronger arm bones than nonswimmers. Stretching out your arms exerts "muscle pull" on the spine, which should help the spine as well as your joints and heart.

Walking and tai chi—which involves weaving, flowing actions with some balancing—are safe for just about everybody, but getting professional advice is always recommended if you have a major health problem.

Yoga

In theory, yogic stretching improves bone strength because you hold the postures for a length of time, which "pulls" on the bones. Muscles are joined to the bones by tendons.

Yoga exercises are done slowly. Once you're at your maximum, you hold the position for at least five slow breaths in and out. Pressure or pull on a bone, whether through gravity (weight) or exertion, tends to cause a degree of stress that then triggers an increase of oxygen and nutrients to the area under pressure. Your body reacts to this type of activity by strengthening the areas that are being stressed.

Yoga confers various advantages.

- Stretching the muscles helps relieve both physical and mental tension.
- Many yoga exercises involve concentration and balance, which should help prevent falls.
- Flexibility improvements make the joints more stable and less rigid, thereby reducing the risk of falls and fractures.
- The emphasis on posture means that the bones in the vertebrae are less likely to collapse because the weak interior part of the spine is not pressured.
- Yoga exercises strengthen the muscles and probably strengthen bones.
- A number of the exercises help the sense of proprioception (awareness of the position of parts of the body without looking at them). This sense tends to weaken as we age and is another factor in falls.
- Mindfulness and concentration training can improve awareness so that you are less careless or impatient, thereby reducing the potential for accidents.
- Willpower is improved.
- Yoga relaxation and meditation techniques help you cope with stress. Relaxing after exercising reduces muscle stiffness caused by a build-up of lactic acid. (Chapter 10 discusses meditation in more detail.)

What to Avoid

- Don't do too much in the beginning. If you're in poor condition, start by walking short distances and do some of the light stretching and strengthening exercises, such as those described below. Once you feel more confident, gradually introduce more difficult activities. Perhaps join a hiking club.
- Bouncing, jerking, prolonged or heavy weight lifting, and skiing are activities I would not recommend to a person with osteoporosis. Exercises that entail extreme arching and bending and lifting heavy loads should be avoided.

- Don't avoid nature walks just because you have osteoporosis. When you walk in the "rough," your ligaments, muscles, and reflexes are more activated and your arms work harder to maintain balance, thereby exercising your back and consequently improving your spine. Walking in natural surroundings is also good for your spirit.
- A dramatic weight loss from overexercising may indicate that the minerals are being pulled out of your bones.
- Don't eat unhealthy foods believing that everything will be burned up from the exercise. When you increase your exercise, you also increase the biochemical activity in the body, including oxidation. Thus, you need quality nutrition, especially plenty of antioxidants in the form of vegetables and fruit.
- When you exercise more, you need to increase your fluid intake but avoid soft drinks and beverages that contain added sugar or aspartame because those substances increase calcium excretion. Water is the best fluid.
- Avoid fad diets. Female athletes and dancers who are under pressure to be thin sometimes experience the cessation of menstrual periods, putting these women at risk for osteoporosis even before menopause.
- Avoid excessive repetition of any single activity that could lead to uneven wearing of joints, causing instability, arthritis, and fractures.

AN EXERCISE PRESCRIPTION

The following exercise prescription has four components: aerobic activities, stretching and strengthening exercises, posture, and relaxation.

I. *Aerobic activities.* Any activity that raises your heart rate, such as a fitness center workout or fast walking, is an aerobic activity. Do such an activity for thirty to forty-five minutes a day, three days a week, preferably alternating the days with stretching and strengthening exercises. You could vary your routine according to the weather and your particular schedule so that you have one exercise-free day. Initially, you may only be able to do ten minutes a day, and it doesn't matter if you take even a few months to build up to thirty minutes a day. If you can't walk for ten minutes, see a doctor before starting.

2. *Stretching and strengthening exercises.* Do these exercises for thirty minutes a day on three separate days. You may need to start with about ten minutes a day.

3. *Posture awareness and improvement.* Make posture part of your daily routine. For some women it's enough to do periodic checks, but others should spend a few minutes each day correcting their sitting and standing postures.

4. *Relaxation.* Being able to relax allows for mental and physical rejuvenation.

Aerobic Fitness

If you can afford it, have a complete fitness examination that includes a blood and heart examination, a treadmill or cycle stress test while being monitored, and a strength and flexibility evaluation.

Planned Exercise   In a planned exercise your pulse rate is quickened and maintained. As long as the heart is sound and there is no disease or disability, the aerobic exercise pulse rate for a sixty-year-old is calculated as follows:

Base number	220
Deduct age	− 60
	160

Training pulse rate is 70 percent of 160, or   112

Depending on one's health, the exercising rate might be 20 percent more or less.

Let's assume you are a healthy sixty-year-old. You can begin the program by walking slowly for five minutes to warm up then walking as fast as you can for, say, five to ten minutes, and then walking slowly for five minutes to cool down. After two or three weeks, add two to five minutes to your walking time and add a few more minutes every two weeks until you're walking fast for twenty minutes (or longer), keeping the five minutes of slow walking at the beginning and the end.

Take your pulse at the beginning of your walk and then again in the middle (when it should be somewhere between 90 and 120 beats a minute, that is, your training rate). At the end of the five-minute cooldown period, the pulse should be within 10 to 15 beats of the starting level. (To test your pulse, the easiest way is to count your rate for ten seconds and then multiply by 6.) For most people the clearest pulse beat to monitor is the carotid artery on the left side of the neck. This area should be gently pressed. Alternatively you can use the wrist (radial) pulse. If taking your pulse is difficult for you, get a demonstration from your health practitioner.

The method I have outlined should be regarded as an approximate guide only. Pulse taking is recommended by most fitness centers throughout the world, but one study has shown that when individuals take their own pulse rate, their evaluation may not be as accurate—as people tend to underestimate the exercising heart rate.[18] The American Council on Exercise recommends a more complex system based on resting heart rate and an individual's functional capacity.[19] A group of medical specialists has also suggested a different and even more complicated formula.[20] In addition, I remind you that the pulse is only one measure of heart and respiratory fitness which is why a professional fitness assessment is recommended before starting an exercise program.

As a general rule, during aerobic exercise you should be able to talk normally and although feeling somewhat "puffed" you should not feel distressed.

Do some aerobic exercise at least three times a week.

Impromptu and Daily-Life Activity   Aim to be as active as possible in your daily life. Keep some walking or running shoes in your car in case you encounter an opportunity to walk or explore. Buy some music that you can dance to at home. On weekends, organize picnics where you can walk or cycle instead of leisurely lunching in a restaurant. Take adventure vacations instead of lazy ones; try a hiking or cycling trip.

ֿst ng and Strengthening Program

beginner exercises I suggest to healthy middle-aged problem with one or two of them, simply leave them some professional help to overcome your particular weak area. If you have difficulty with a number of them or if you are disabled, get professional advice on ways of strengthening and mobilizing your body to your capacity.

It's not easy to suggest the appropriate level for each individual, but if you don't feel a stretch or the muscles working, you won't improve. Conversely, you should not feel pain.

If you just stick to these exercises year after year, you'll get bored; your body and mind enjoy new challenges. Find books at your library or bookstore, see a physiotherapist or a yoga teacher, or join a gym. It's also good to have a variety of options, especially if you have an injury or some arthritic pain in a few joints, but there is usually no reason why you can't exercise the nonpainful areas.

The plan suggests a selection of the stretching and strengthening exercises for thirty minutes a day three times a week. You may want to read aloud and tape-record these directions, pausing between each sentence because these exercises are done slowly.

Simple Warm-Ups

1. Standing with legs apart, swing from side to side with your arms loose, turning your head as you swing.
2. Do half knee bends with feet together, gently swinging your arms backward and forward.
3. Stand with legs apart, arms bent, fingertips on the shoulders; bring the elbows together in front of you, letting the head drop forward; then take the elbows up and back, making circles with the elbows and letting the head drop back.

Do about ten rounds of each warm-up, then walk around the room high on the balls of your feet.

Basic Tips

- If you do stretching and mobilizing exercises slowly and rhythmically, you are unlikely to do any damage.
- Where breathing is not specifically mentioned, aim to breathe slowly and evenly. Holding the breath is not good during exercising; if you find yourself doing so, gently exhale through the mouth.
- Always breathe in through the nose. You are aiming for a slow, unforced rhythmical breathing pattern, which is generally more easily achieved if you breathe out through the nose. When I jog, I have to breathe in through the mouth, otherwise I don't get enough oxygen.
- It is said that a person is born with only so many breaths, so if you habitually breathe very quickly, you will use them up!
- In yoga, we say that you should have the forehead smooth and calm and have a little half-smile on your lips while you are exercising. Smiling is the best exercise for your face.
- If one side of your body is weaker or stiffer, it is advisable to do double the activity on that side so that you balance the muscles and joints.

(a) Thigh Strengthening

1. Standing upright, take a small step forward with the right foot, coming up on the balls of both feet, hands loosely clasped behind the back.
2. Keeping the back straight, bend both knees and lower yourself about 4 inches toward the floor.
3. Hold for ten breaths.
4. Repeat with the left leg in front.

(b) Hip Strengthener and Balancer

1. Stand upright, looking straight ahead, hands on the waist.
2. Bring the right knee up as high as possible toward the chest.
3. Keeping the knee up and the shoulders to the front, take the right leg to the side.

4. Hold in that position for ten breaths. (Perhaps three breaths is all you can manage at first.)
5. Repeat with the other leg.

(c) Thigh and Knee Stretch

1. Stand upright, looking straight ahead.
2. Bend your left leg behind you, grasping the left foot with both hands.
3. Pull the left foot toward the buttocks, trying to get the left knee in line with the right knee without bending the body forward.
4. Hold for five breaths in and out.
5. Repeat with the other leg.

(d) Spine Stretch with Ankle Circles

1. Stand upright, looking straight ahead.
2. Slowly bring the left knee up toward the chest, holding it with both hands.
3. Do five slow ankle circles each direction with the left ankle.
4. Repeat with the right leg.

You will notice that the above exercises work the balance muscles located on the outer part of the legs. These balance exercises also strengthen the hip joint.

(e) Neck and Shoulder Movements

1. Lie on the floor on your right side, right arm straight and slightly in front, head resting on the floor, right leg straight, left leg bent with the left knee on the floor in front of you.
2. Slowly take the left arm backward in a circle, following your left hand with your eyes. The aim is to have the left arm relaxed and to make a low, wide circle. Your head turns but stays on the floor or on the right arm, whichever is more comfortable.
3. Do ten circles, then repeat on the other side.

Once you are used to the movement, coordinate the exercise with your breathing. As you are taking the upper arm back, the chest expands and you should be breathing in. When the arm is coming forward, you breathe out.

(f) Spinal Twist

1. Sit on the floor, legs straight in front.
2. Place both hands on the floor on the right side of the thigh.
3. Slowly raise your right hand to shoulder level and take the right arm as far as you can behind you, watching the hand with your eyes, without straining the neck.
4. When you've twisted as far as you can, place the right hand on the floor behind you, keep looking to the right, and take five gentle breaths in and out. The aim is to get the shoulders in line with the middle of the legs. The right arm is working and there is pressure in the right shoulder blade area.
5. Lift both hands off the floor and slowly turn your body back to the center.
6. Repeat on the left side.

This stretch mobilizes the middle part of the back and the shoulders. You can do a similar twist while sitting on a straight-backed chair.

(g) Toning Upper Arms (Triceps) and Wrists

1. Sit on the floor, your back close to a solid footstool or the base of a low armchair, legs bent and feet flat on the floor.
2. Bend your arms backward so that your hands rest on the top of the footstool with the fingers forward.
3. Cross your left leg over the right leg.
4. Slowly push up with your arms until they are straight, hold the position for one breath in and out, then gently lower down so that your bottom almost touches the floor.
5. Repeat twenty times and then again with the right leg over the left. (Initially you may only be able to do five!)

(h) Arm Strengthening (Modified Push-Ups)

1. Kneel on all fours, with your knees on a soft rug; position the knees so that you're resting on the thigh end of the kneecaps.
2. Bend the elbows, letting the head drop forward and down so that the chin almost touches the floor.

3. Push up, puffing out through the mouth.
4. Repeat at least ten times.

(i) Upper Body Toner

1. Lie on your stomach, feet on the floor, elbows bent, fingers touching, and chin resting on your fingers.
2. Breathing in, slowly lift your upper body as you count to five, keeping your chin on your fingers; feet stay on the floor.
3. Breathing out, slowly lower your body back to the floor.
4. Repeat three times.

Lying on your tummy for long periods is not good for your lower back. After any exercise like this one, come up onto your knees, let your buttocks go down toward your heels, keep your body in a low position, aiming to put the forehead on the floor, and stretch the arms in front of you with your hands on the floor. Maintain the stretch for five slow breaths, then relax the elbows and stay with the head down for a further five slow breaths. Sit up slowly.

(j) Sit-Downs

1. Sit with knees bent, feet flat on the floor.
2. Tuck your chin down to your upper chest and slowly curl down until your head is on the floor, making sure that your chin stays down and your lower abdomen does the work.

If this exercise strains your back, start with a pillow on the floor behind you so that you don't have to go all the way down.

(k) Pelvic Rock

1. Lie on your back, knees bent, feet flat on the floor.
2. As you breathe out, push the lower back into the floor, tighten the buttocks so that they are slightly off the floor, and suck the abdomen in tightly, picturing the navel touching the spine.
3. Breathe in, relax, and let your back come off the floor and your hips roll gently forward.
4. Repeat ten times.

Make sure you're working at pulling the abdomen flat as you breathe out and relaxing your lower back as you breathe in.

(l) Modified Sit-Ups

1. Lie on your back, knees bent, feet flat on the floor, elbows bent, hands behind your neck.
2. Suck in your abdomen, bring your upper body up so that your shoulder blades are a few inches off the floor as you are breathing out and squeezing the abdomen down. Put your mind to your abdomen, and look up to the ceiling so that you are not curling the neck.
3. Smoothly lower the body down. Relax, breath in.
4. Repeat at least ten times.

You can progress to more difficult sit-ups as your abdominal muscles strengthen and your back becomes more flexible.

Do not do sit-ups if you have a serious or constant lower back problem unless you are monitored by a health professional.

Apart from looking unattractive, a saggy, protruding abdomen puts stress on the back; but a little roundness is healthy.

(m) Hip and Side Twist

1. Lie on the floor on your back, legs straight.
2. Bend your right leg, so that the foot is flat on the floor next to your left knee.
3. Put your right toes under your left knee and bend your arms so that the elbows are level with the shoulders and the palms are facing upward (hands flat on the floor).
4. Slowly let your right leg drop over to the left side, releasing your left hand so that you can use finger pressure to push the right knee toward the floor while the right elbow stays on the floor.
5. Relax, imagining that with each breath out your body and legs are becoming soft.
6. After five breaths in and out, come up and repeat on the other side.

Repeat at least twice, aiming to relax into the exercise without using force. This exercise is also good for the upper back and shoulders. You will probably feel that the muscles around your armpits are very tight. These muscles help to keep your breasts from sagging, but if the muscles are not flexible, the shoulders tend to pull forward so that the back is hunched over.

(n) Tummy and Buttock Trimmer

1. Lie on your back, knees bent, feet apart and flat on the floor, and bend your arms so that the elbows are level with the shoulders and the palms are facing upward (hands flat on the floor).
2. Lift up your buttocks without arching the back, keeping the shoulders on the floor.
3. Squeeze the buttock muscles and suck in the lower abdomen, picturing the navel touching the spine.
4. As you squeeze and tighten, exhale out. Your thighs will move a little in the process, but remember that you're concentrating on the area between the waist and the upper thighs.
5. Relax, breathe in, and let the body drop down a little.
6. Repeat ten times.

This exercise also helps the bladder and the back.

(o) Side Lift-Ups

1. Lie on your right side, right elbow bent, forearm on the floor in front of you, left arm lightly resting on your left side, legs straight, left foot on top of the right foot, feet straight in front.
2. Keeping the right forearm on the floor and using it as a support, lift the middle of the body off the floor so that you're in a straight sloping line from the head to the feet. The aim is to lift the body rather than push up from the bent right arm. You should feel the right side of the body working.
3. Do twenty lifts and then repeat on the other side. (It may take a few weeks before you can do twenty!)

This exercise strengthens the side of the body, but it is also very good for spinal strength and stability because there are not many exercises that work the spine in this way.

(p) Forward Stretch, for Mobilizing the Hip Joint

1. Sit on the floor with your legs crossed, right leg in front.
2. Take a deep breath in; as you breathe out, stretch your arms in front of you with the hands on the floor. Pull in your abdomen, let your head drop down, and fold your arms in front of you.
3. Stay down for five breaths, feeling that you're melting down with each breath out. Do not use force, as that can strain the lower back and legs.
4. Slowly come up and uncross your legs.
5. Repeat with the left leg in front.

(q) Back Extension: The Cobra

1. Lie on your stomach, feet on the floor, hands on the floor under your shoulders, fingers to the front.
2. As you breathe in, lift up the upper body, pushing down with the arms while keeping the hips on the floor. Keep the chin level and thrust the chest forward. Do not attempt to straighten the arms unless you are very flexible.
3. Come up to your discomfort (but not painful) level; do five slow exhales through the mouth and slowly lower the body to the floor.
4. Repeat once.

This exercise is especially good for strengthening the lower spine; it also strengthens the arms.

(r) Side and Leg Stretch

1. Sit on the floor, left leg bent behind you to the left side, right leg stretching out to the right side in front of you.
2. Place your hands on either side of your right thigh.

3. Take a deep breath in, feel tall; as you breathe out, pull in your abdomen and stretch over to the right as far as you can without overstraining. Then let your head drop down.
4. Focus on your breath and feel that you are relaxing over and down with each breath out. Stay down for five breaths in and out.
5. Slowly come up and repeat on the other side.

This exercise can also be done with the legs stretched out to either side.

(s) Back Mobilizer: The Cat

1. Kneel on your hands and knees, arms straight, hands level with the shoulders, fingers pointing forward.
2. Breathing out, drop your head downward and pull your abdomen up and in as far as possible, arching your back upward at the same time, picturing the navel touching the spine.
3. Breathing in, lift your head up and smoothly rock the bottom upward, trying to get movement in the lower back area.
4. Repeat ten times.

In this exercise you're working hard as you breathe out and relaxing as you breathe in.

(t) Hip Strengthener and Mobilizer

1. Kneel on your hands and knees.
2. Slowly straighten your right leg behind you with the foot off the floor and level with your body.
3. Keeping the right foot up as high as possible, slowly bring the right leg in an arc, aiming to get the foot level with the waist. This movement is very uncomfortable and is difficult for most people.
4. Hold for ten breaths, or as long as you can.
5. Repeat with the other leg.

(u) Hip Rock

1. Sit on the floor, legs in front.
2. Bend the right leg and clasp the right foot with both hands, aiming to put the right foot inside the left elbow or as far as you can.

3. Cradle both arms around the right leg and gently rock your whole body from side to side as if rocking a baby.

4. Do ten rocks, and then repeat with the other leg.

(v) Hamstring Stretches

1. Sit on the floor, with knees bent outward, feet toward each other.
2. Hold the right foot or the lower right leg with the right hand; the left hand stays on the floor slightly behind you.
3. Slowly straighten the right leg upward and outward as far as you can.
4. Hold for five breaths.
5. Do at least three repetitions of this with each leg.
6. You can use a band around your foot to make it easier.

If the muscles at the back of the leg are stiff, you will usually have lower back problems because these muscles are connected to the hip.

(w) Rowing (Without the Oars and the Boat!)

1. Sit on the floor, legs in front, hands on the knees.
2. Let the hands smoothly glide down your legs as you breathe out and suck in the abdomen. Don't jerk or overstrain.
3. Slowly come back upright as you breathe in.
4. Do at least ten repetitions.

(x) Knee Circling

1. Lie on your back and bring both knees up to your chest, clasping them with your hands.
2. Give yourself some hugs and then little rocks from side to side.
3. Do three knee circles each way while you are still holding your knees.

(y) Quick Relaxation and Rejuvenation: Yoga Nidra

1. Lie flat on the floor, face upward, legs slightly apart, feet dropping to the sides, arms slightly out from the body, palms facing upward.

2. Push the lower back into the floor and then relax.
3. Push the back of the neck down toward the floor and then relax.
4. Close your eyes, have a little smile on the lips, and relax your fore-head and the muscles of your face.
5. Watch your breath as it gently flows in and out through the nostrils.
6. Visualize a soft glowing light and picture yourself breathing in that light, making your mind clear and calm, your body light and soft.
7. Feel that you're so light that you can hardly feel the floor beneath you.
8. Keep picturing the light for a few minutes.
9. Take a few deeper breaths in and out, breathing in energy into your light, soft body.
10. Open your eyes, give a big stretch upward, bring your knees up to the chest, give yourself some hugs, and then lie on your side for five breaths before you sit up.

Most people find that lying straight as in this exercise for a short period of time is very refreshing, but if you do it for too long, your back may get uncomfortable or you may feel drowsy.

(z) Body Circling

1. Stand upright, feet apart, arms relaxed but stretched above the head.
2. Do three wide circles each way with the arms and body.

Posture

You may have heard that women can lose up to 6 inches in height because of osteoporosis. The only way you'll become 6 inches shorter as you age is if a portion of your legs is amputated, if you have extremely bad posture, or if you have an extremely frail body.

Of course, some elderly people with severe osteoporosis experience a collapse in part of the spine, which generally causes the head to drop forward and the upper body to slump over. Good postural habits together with strong muscles gained by exercise, however, can offset even severe osteoporosis. In fact, many of my elderly patients do not have a dowagers hump, and they sit and walk with a relatively straight spine. Habitual good posture may even prevent spinal collapse. If you look at a picture of the spine, you will see that there is not much bone and muscle protection around the part of the spine that faces into the body; therefore, if your spine is already curving, it is more likely to collapse if the bones are osteoporotic.

The combination of good posture and strong muscles has distinct advantages.

- Both help prevent harmful changes in the body's supporting structures, such as wearing down the inner portions of the spine.
- Healthy muscles retain both elasticity and strength so that, for example, the shoulders are not pulled forward. Even excessively tight muscles at the back of the legs can affect your posture.
- Strong abdominal muscles prevent an exaggerated curvature of the lower back, avoiding compensatory changes in the upper spine.
- A relaxed upright body allows for breathing efficiency and better circulation.
- You feel more confident in your daily activities and in emergencies when you need to react.
- You'll recover more quickly if you're injured or require surgery.
- Your whole appearance is positive. People with bad posture often appear downcast and tired.
- Good posture and healthy muscles make you look ten years younger. Test it for yourself. Stand in front of a full-length mirror and let your body sag, with your head drooping forward. Then stand upright with the chin level and add a little half smile.

Of course, you shouldn't attempt to be rigidly upright either, because that position will lead to backache and muscle stress. When you feel really tired from long periods of sitting or standing, take a short break: lie down on a firm surface, go for a short walk, or stretch. Even just twisting sideways in your chair will help.

Remind yourself throughout the day to keep the spine upright, the chin level, and the shoulders relaxed and visualize that you are breathing in light and energy. Feel that your body is tall and that you are gently lifting upward from the middle of the body rather than trying to force your shoulders backward. If you feel tense, try gently rocking backward and forward or slowly turning your head from side to side. Clasp your hands behind your back and squeeze your shoulder blades together for a few seconds. Do occasional mirror checks. Is your head tilted to one side? Does one shoulder droop? Are your hips both at the same level? One of the best ways of improving your posture is to become aware of it.

Here are some specific ways to check and improve your posture:

- Using two straps, tie one under the armpits and the other around the waist, not too tightly. I use thick, soft webbing (available at camping stores) and sew two "D" buckles onto one end. These can also be used for leg stretches.
- Sit in a straight-backed chair.
- Push a narrow, wooden curtain rod through both straps so that the rod runs along your spine and rests on the chair. The lower end of the rod lightly touches your lower spine and the upper portion just touches the back of your head. At first you may feel somewhat uncomfortable. Don't worry if your head does not touch the rod because you may have a structural problem that prevents this position.
- Use a mirror so that you can turn your head to check that you are at least almost upright, or get someone to check you.
- Do not lift your chin to tilt your head back to touch the rod, because that puts pressure on the back of the neck and is bad for your throat.
- In this position, aim for an even breathing rhythm with the shoulders relaxed.
- Feel that you are gently lifting up from the rib cage and that the top of the head is rising while the chin stays level.
- Imagine that you are using your breath to make your body light and tall.

- Sit this way for a few minutes every day and do mirror checks of yourself. You will gradually appreciate what it feels like to be relaxed and upright. Instead of flopping into a chair and slumping, sit up rather than sit down. In time, you will be able to get into a good postural position without the use of the straps and rod.

Another way of testing your posture is to use a wall.

- Stand without shoes with your heels slightly out from the wall. The back of your hair should lightly touch the wall (with your chin level). The shoulder blade area and buttocks should also touch the wall.
- Place your hand behind your lower back, palm facing the wall, and suck in your lower abdomen so that the small of the back lightly touches your hand. Then release the hand.
- Relax your shoulders and hold the position for about five relaxed breaths.
- Repeat the procedure at least three times and then do a mirror check of yourself.

Meditation stools are excellent spine straighteners, and most people automatically get into a good posture when using them. It's okay to have a slight forward tilt as long as you are not hunched over. A suitable size for people who are average or above-average height and build is 18½ inches across, 7½ inches from back to front, 5½ inches front height, and 6½ inches back height.

Small people would be more comfortable in a much lower position. You can also make a meditation stool by taking a small coffee table and simply cutting off the legs of the table until you find the right height and angle for yourself. Yoga centers and catalogs also sell meditation stools.

When you are sitting or standing for long periods, alternately tighten and relax your abdominal muscles. With each exhalation, picture your navel touching your spine, and then relax as you breathe in. When you breathe out in this way, you are making your abdominal muscles work and are helping your posture. During your work day, you can do a less forceful version of this exercise by keeping the breath even and relaxed, maintaining a little half smile, and gently holding in the abdomen. In other words, you can be doing a posture and abdominal exercise without anyone else knowing.

Remember also that your feet affect your posture. If your shoes wear down unevenly or if you have a foot problem, get professional help immediately to correct or modify the fault.

Modern Furniture and Its Effect on Posture   The main problem with furniture in the home, and often at work, is that it is rarely adjustable. Mass-produced furniture is designed for the "average" person, so it probably suits about half the adult population, or one person per household.

Some yoga teachers say that as far as our backs and hips are concerned, furniture is the worst invention. Even people in developing countries have better posture than we do. Poor people in India, for example, who habitually sit on the floor, generally walk and sit in a good postural position and do not have the extent of hip fractures compared with, say, wealthier Indians who live in Singapore.

Aside from checking yourself, start observing other people and picturing how good-looking they would appear if only they had an upright, relaxed body, and a little half smile!

Doing a wide variety of activities and maintaining correct postural positions will help keep your joints stable, strong, and flexible.

You may want to learn how to sit comfortably on the floor. Sitting in lotus or similar positions puts pressure on the cartilage around the outer edges of the hip joints. Consequently, there is resistance over the whole area of the joint for at least part of the day, which should lead to more stable hip joints. Uneven wearing of joint tissue is a problem, especially in arthritis, because it causes instability when standing and walking as well as the tendency to fall and sustain a fracture. Instability of the hip also affects the spine and neck because your body tries to compensate to keep you upright.

I suggest that you start sitting cross-legged on the floor for a few minutes each day. In my yoga classes the students do lots of leg flexibility exercises and practice sitting on the floor on the edge of a large pillow, a bolster, or even a book. Sitting this way is easier and more comfortable than other positions and is an ideal way of sitting, because your legs form a stable triangular base and you can gently rock or move to avoid becoming rigid. It is also a good posture for those who practice deep meditation, because some meditators become somewhat anxious about falling, sleeping, or slumping when sitting in a chair. The main advantage of sitting cross-legged is that it is an excellent stretch for the hips.

If you have a knee problem, you may need to use a small pillow under the knee or sit cross-legged with a pillow at your back and under both knees. It's okay to lean forward slightly as long as your neck and back are not hunched over.

Relaxation

A very comfortable position for relaxing is to lie on a firm surface with a low cushion to support your neck and a very large cushion under the knees.

Relaxation and exercise complement each other. After exercise, most people have much better quality relaxation; the relaxation in turn reduces the buildup of lactic acid that follows physical activity. Interestingly, blood levels of lactic acid are also relatively high in people who are mentally stressed, which is one reason your muscles can feel tight and sore even though you haven't exercised. If you feel really tense, it is not possible to relax, but some stretching exercises will help reduce physical and mental tension.

Relaxation has other benefits as well. It

- Reduces anxiety
- Facilitates rest and sleep
- Reduces physical pain and discomfort
- Enables better thinking and concentration
- Rejuvenates
- Improves relationships

Activity regenerates; inactivity degenerates. Although ideally you should have built up your bones, connective tissue, and muscles from infancy onward, a brisk walking program alone can have beneficial effects on the mind and body of even very elderly nonexercisers. Be in constant touch with your best two doctors: your right leg and your left leg.

Each person makes decisions every day that affect health and quality of life, and one such decision is the choice between an active or a sedentary lifestyle. If you choose to be sedentary, you have selected a course that is a risk factor for disease. A prescription for exercise (if followed) is not a guarantee that you will be forever young and free of disease, but it does decrease your chance of developing a number of serious degenerative diseases, becoming depressed, aging prematurely, and becoming dependent on others. My observations also indicate that habitual exercisers seem to have a more positive attitude and recover more effectively from illness and injury than sedentary people.

It's never too late to benefit from an increase in physical activity; you can slowly improve flexibility, strength, and endurance. A prescription for exercise is a prescription for quality of life.

CHAPTER EIGHT

Bone-Friendly Nutrients

*B*ones require *all* the forty-five essential nutrients, and *essential* means that you need to consume these nutrients because the body can't make them. In animal experiments, a diet devoid of *any* essential nutrient, such as vitamin E or manganese, will result in osteoporosis. Thus, a focus solely on calcium is not beneficial for bones or general health.

A U.S. trial comparing the results of calcium alone with the results of calcium plus trace elements showed that the addition of trace elements was helpful for bones, whereas calcium alone was not.[1] One British medical researcher studied the nutritional profiles of osteoporotic women and found that none had low calcium levels, but they were low in many other nutrients associated with bone development.[2] Of course, I am not minimizing that calcium is a major bone nutrient and that some women may have benefited from a calcium-rich diet and calcium supplements. In fact, over 40,000 scientific papers have been published on various aspects of calcium.

To have healthy bones, however, you do need to digest and absorb the various nutrients as well as to not lose too many nutrients through the urine or feces. Sulfur-rich proteins, fat, phytates, oxalates, salt, and caffeine increase calcium excretion, whereas B vitamins decrease calcium excretion.[3] (Chapter 6 also covers aspects of interactions and excretion of nutrients.)

Sometimes during menopause, with all the emphasis on hormones, bones, and calcium, you may be misled into disregarding other important nutrients and functions of the body. For instance, your heart needs to pump the blood to carry nutrients and oxygen, and your blood vessels need to have the right mix of strength and elasticity. These important health topics are addressed in chapter 9.

THERE IS NO SUBSTITUTE FOR GOOD NUTRITION

The best way of getting good nutrition is to eat a variety of foods in as natural a state as possible. Each plant contains up to 500 different compounds, including nutrients, antioxidants, chemicals that help prevent cancer, oils, hormone-like compounds, digestive aids, and starches that provide energy. No supplement can surpass nature. The following nutrients are key to bone health.

- Vitamin K is lower in women with osteoporosis than in women without osteoporosis.[4] The best food source of vitamin K is green leafy vegetables; this vitamin is also produced in the intestines by bacteria. If intestinal health is defective, however, this natural conversion may be impeded.
- Dietary vitamin C, but not vitamin C from supplements, was correlated with higher bone mineral density at the femur (the narrow part of the upper leg).[5] Fruits and vegetables are the best dietary sources of vitamin C, and they are rich in flavonoids, which may also be important for bone health.
- Smokers with a low intake of both vitamin E and vitamin C intake had a 4.9-fold higher risk for hip fracture.[6]
- Fruit and vegetable consumption has been linked to improved bone health.[7] A high vegetable intake provides potassium, which reduces urinary excretion of calcium.[8]
- Isoflavones (plant estrogens) in soy and other foods are possibly helpful in maintaining bone health.[9] Two isoflavones in particular

(genistein and genistin) have produced bone-building effects in animal studies.

- Zinc, copper, magnesium, manganese, boron, vitamin C, vitamin B_6, and folic acid are specifically linked to bone health.[10]
- Trace elements such as boron may help bone quality because they activate enzymes involved in producing the connective tissue that forms the structure of bone.[11] (The basic role of enzymes in the body is to activate reactions; without them, reactions would not occur or would not occur effectively.)
- A study showed that animal protein, compared with soy protein, had about the same amount of calcium, but the calcium excretion rate was about 50 percent higher with the animal protein diet. (See table 8.1.) In elderly women with a recent osteoporotic hip fracture, the addition of a protein supplement along with other nutrients produced a better result than consuming other nutrients alone.[12] This finding doesn't mean that all osteoporotic patients would benefit from protein supplementation, but some elderly people (and vegans) who have small appetites or restricted diets may be marginally deficient in protein, and bones need adequate, though not excessive, protein.
- Lactose intolerance may be relatively high in infants, and then it apparently decreases and re-emerges later in life in a significant

TABLE 8.1 **Protein and Calcium Excretion**		
	Animal Protein (mg/day)	*Soy Protein (mg/day)*
Calcium intake	447	440
Calcium excretion	150	103

Source: Adapted from N. A. Breslau, L. Brinkley and C. Y. C. Pak, "Relationship of Animal Protein-Rich Diet to Kidney Stone Formation and Calcium Metabolism," *Journal of Clinical Endocrinology and Metabolism* 66 (1988): 140–46.

proportion of postmenopausal women. Because the sugar in milk (lactose) becomes nondigestible, it irritates the digestive tract, causing diarrhea and reducing nutrient absorption. Consequently, lactose intolerance is linked to osteoporosis. Dairy foods can therefore cause bone weakness if you are lactose intolerant. Furthermore, the highest rates of osteoporosis occur in countries with the highest intake of calcium.[13] In these osteoporotic countries, dairy foods are a common source of calcium. Be aware that anything that causes digestive irritation or diarrhea is likely to be harmful to you.

- Women taking hormones are more likely to have nutrient deficiencies and imbalances than women not taking hormones. These nutrient deficiencies and imbalances are likely to contribute to impaired bone production. International data show that arm fractures have increased dramatically among women aged thirty-five to sixty-four years, becoming six times more common in countries with the highest rates of hormone takers. Few older women take hormones, and there is no lasting protection among older women who have the most risk of hip fractures. In contrast, maintaining adequate nutritional status is a key requirement for health and safely improves serum bone ALP (alkaline phosphatase) activity and bone formation.[14] (ALP is an enzyme.)

IMPORTANT BONE NUTRIENTS

Essential Fatty Acids

Essential fatty acids increase calcium uptake in the intestines and reduce the calcium excreted in the urine. A combination of fish oil and evening primrose oil (providing eicosapentanoic acid and gamma-linolenic acid) given to elderly women showed no change in the lumbar spine and a 1.3 percent increase in the femoral neck, compared with placebo that showed decreases of 3.2 percent and 2.1 percent. Both groups were given 600 milligrams calcium daily.[15]

A biochemical study showed that fish oil produced indications of bone improvements. Evening primrose oil alone had no significant effects, but when combined with fish oil, it boosted the activity of the fish oil in respect to calcium metabolism.[16] Other studies confirm that elderly patients with osteoporosis tend to have increased calcifications in soft tissues, particularly the arteries and the kidneys. Because fish oil is effective in preventing kidney stone formation, this finding suggests that fish oil helps calcium get to where it is needed in the body and this is supported by my clinical experience.

Vitamin E

It is known that vitamin E deficiency causes osteoporosis in rats. An animal study suggests that vitamin E may protect against oxidation in cartilage and bone cells, thereby helping with their growth.[17] In my own case, when I was diagnosed with osteoporosis I analyzed my diet and assessed that it was marginally deficient in vitamin E (because I had been on a very low fat diet). I took 500 IU (800 milligrams) of vitamin E daily, along with other supplements, and went from moderate osteoporosis to normal bones in one year. I also dropped the low-fat diet and began eating avocado, nuts, seeds, and olive oil in moderate quantities.

I now give all my osteoporosis patients a supplement containing 500 milligrams fish oil, 500 milligrams evening primrose oil, and 34 milligrams vitamin E. When I omitted this combination supplement from my initial osteoporosis program, the patients did not do as well.

Standard Dosage   Take one capsule before breakfast and one before bed, taken with other supplements as indicated in appendix IV. If you can afford it, discuss with your practitioner whether double this dose may be even more beneficial for you.

Magnesium

Magnesium is essential for calcium and vitamin D metabolism, for regulating parathyroid hormone, and for alkaline phosphatase, an enzyme involved in forming calcium crystals in bone.

In one study, almost three-fourths of a group of thirty-one women who took between 250 and 750 milligrams of magnesium daily for two years showed bone density increases of 1 to 8 percent, whereas seventeen other women who refused the supplement lost 1 to 3 percent of their bone density during the same period.[18] In another trial, magnesium supplementation of 250 milligrams daily appeared to prevent fractures as well as result in a significant increase in bone density.[19]

Some medical researchers have claimed that magnesium deficiency is responsible for osteoporosis and that this deficiency causes abnormal crystal formation in bones.[20] Animal studies confirm that low magnesium intake during growth can alter the quality and quantity of bone, suggesting that magnesium deprivation may contribute to the development of osteoporosis.

Other researchers state that treating postmenopausal osteoporosis with estrogen and calcium disregards the likelihood that an excess of these two remedies may increase magnesium requirements.[21] Because primary postmenopausal osteoporosis is predominantly due to demineralization of trabecular bone, there is no justification for calcium megadosing in postmenopausal women.[22]

A dietary program emphasizing magnesium instead of calcium increased bone mineral density by 11 percent in postmenopausal women on hormone replacement therapy.[23]

Magnesium overdosing, however, can cause problems such as diarrhea, high blood pressure, and irregular heartbeat. Magnesium is also used in some antacids, so always study the labels of any type of supplement or medication and check with your health practitioner if you are on pharmaceuticals. Table 8.2 lists foods rich in magnesium.

Boron

Boron is a trace element. It is poisonous in large doses, as is the case with all trace elements. It does not, however, seem to accumulate in the body to any measurable extent,[24] and it has a number of benefits.

Boron helps the body make estrogen and testosterone; therefore, it is ideal for postmenopausal women but not for menstruating women or

TABLE 8.2 **Foods Rich in Magnesium**	
Magnesium-rich foods	*Magnesium (mg/100 g)*
Cocoa (dry powder)	420
Basil (powder)	410
Cumin	390
Wheat germ	336
Curry powder	284
Almonds	270
Pine nuts	268
Cashews	267
Soya beans	235
Brazil nuts	225

Note: Many other foods—including grains, legumes, and green leafy vegetables—are quite good sources of magnesium.

women on HRT. One report suggests that boron appears capable of producing an estrogenic effect without exposing the body to dangerous amounts of estrogen.[25]

Some researchers suggest that boron may help alleviate menopausal symptoms, but any improvement in estrogen status would be extremely weak. I have not found this effect powerful enough to offset symptoms in my patients.

Boron's role in osteoporosis is associated with interactions, notably with magnesium. It reduces urinary calcium excretion, alleviates vitamin D deficiency, and is involved in the conversion of cholesterol to both vitamin D and steroid hormones. Adverse effects of fluoride may be offset by boron. A maximum dosage for this effect would be 10 to 12 milligrams a day.

An international comparison suggests that the prevalence of arthritis is inversely proportional to the level of boron in soil and subsequently the food supply.[26] A small double-blind pilot study showed that boron offset pain, swelling, and stiffness in 50 to 71 percent of arthritis patients, compared with 10 to 30 percent of those on placebo.[27]

A diet very low in boron leads to a faster rate of aging, but moderate amounts extend lifespan and may improve brain function. Two human studies on boron deprivation caused changes that could be construed as being detrimental to bone formation and maintenance.[28] It has been suggested that boron does not help bones unless accompanied by physical activity, which again emphasizes the importance of combining a healthy diet and lifestyle.

A well-known boron researcher indicates a minimal intake of 13 milligrams a day, but diets low in fruits, vegetables, nuts, and legumes may not supply even this amount.[29] In some parts of the world, the diet contains as much as 41 milligrams of boron daily with apparently no harmful consequences. Dried fruits such as raisins, dried parsley, and wine are particularly good sources of boron.[30]

Boron is essential for plants; plants such as cauliflower with a boron deficiency develop cavities in their stems (osteoporotic vegetables!). There is currently some debate as to whether boron should be officially declared an essential nutrient for humans.

With nearly all my osteoporosis patients, I prescribe a 3 milligrams boron supplement combined with 125 milligrams magnesium taken before breakfast and before bed (3 milligrams is about $\frac{1}{1,000}$ of a teaspoon).

When I used magnesium alone, patients' bones did not respond as effectively as in those patients who took the magnesium plus the boron. This finding needs to be verified on a larger number of patients.

Zinc

Zinc is essential for human growth. It affects taste and smell and is a cofactor for hormones and bone enzymes as well as vitamin D. A zinc deficiency causes problems in bone matrix formation.[31] American and Australian diets (and presumably those elsewhere) are typically low in zinc. Major dietary surveys of adults indicate that the majority consume a level considerably lower than the recommended dietary intake. Women on the pill and HRT are known to have reduced zinc levels.

Elderly people with low appetites and women on hormone therapy are likely to benefit from zinc supplementation. Anyone with poor nutrition may also benefit from zinc supplementation, but if your diet is deficient in zinc, it is also likely to be deficient in other nutrients.

Manganese

Manganese is needed for bone mineralization and connective tissue. In one study, women on HRT were found to have low manganese levels.[32] A study of osteoporotic women showed that blood manganese levels were only 25 percent of age-matched women who did not have osteoporosis. Osteoporotic women on HRT may have an even worse manganese status, which may be why women on HRT have a higher incidence of arthritis and why HRT is not generally successful for improving bones.

The calcium citrate supplement I prescribe also contains a small amount of zinc, manganese, and silica, plus vitamin K and vitamin D.

Copper

Copper is a cofactor of an enzyme involved in collagen fibers; it also interacts with other trace elements.[33] Copper deficiency in humans and animals is associated with bone fragility due to defective cross-links in collagen (bone protein). This deficiency results in bones that are brittle and lack toughness.[34] It may also explain the folk remedy of using copper for joint problems.

Copper levels may be high in women who take HRT, however, and copper levels in water may also be high where copper pipes are used. I have never recommended supplemental copper to my patients, although it might be helpful for those women who have a known deficiency.

Silicon

At lease five animal studies have demonstrated that a silicon-deficient diet causes abnormal bones. The primary role of silicon is thought to be in the bone matrix because it is found in glycosaminoglycans (connective tissue). Researchers suggest that silicon appears to affect the initiation and rate of bone mineralization.[35] Herbalists often prescribe horsetail herb (*Equisetum arvense*) as a silicon supplement.

Other Trace Elements

Molybdenum, vanadium, strontium, gallium, nickel, rubidium, platinum, and even tin may also be linked to skeletal development.[36] Until more is known about all the trace elements, it might be wise to consume a wide variety of plant foods and avoid megadosing on calcium, which may inhibit the absorption of some essential trace elements.

Vitamin K

Vitamin K is needed for bone structure. Minerals get deposited within the bone matrix (a network of protein fibers). Vitamin K supplements may be helpful in treating osteoporosis and fractures because people with osteoporosis frequently have low levels of this vitamin.[37] Vitamin K deficiency in animals causes a large increase in urinary calcium excretion.

Pyridoxine (Vitamin B$_6$)

Deficiency of vitamin B$_6$ produces osteoporosis in animals. Pyridoxine is also a cofactor in bone structure (collagen metabolism) and is also useful for breaking down homocysteine, a natural by-product of protein metabolism, which apparently promotes osteoporosis.[38]

Folic Acid (Vitamin B$_9$)

Vitamin B$_9$ also breaks down homocysteine, which is not only implicated in osteoporosis but in other degenerative aging problems. Both vitamins B$_6$ and B$_9$ deficiencies tend to be more prevalent in HRT users than in nonusers.[39]

Vitamin B$_{12}$

Vitamin B$_{12}$ is known to stimulate human bone cells, and a deficiency (pernicious anemia) is a risk factor for osteoporosis.[40] Furthermore, vitamin B$_{12}$ breaks down homocysteine, a problem compound in human aging. As we age, vitamin B$_{12}$ absorption also becomes somewhat unreliable.

Vitamin D

Vitamin D deficiency is fairly common among the elderly due to lack of sunlight, low dietary intake, poor absorption, or metabolism problems. Table 8.3 lists foods rich in vitamin D. Supplementation has shown modest improvements in bone mineral density and reduced fracture risk. Vitamin D is required for intestinal calcium absorption, but it has to be converted to a biologically active form to be usable by the body. Magnesium and boron are thought to help this conversion.

In elderly women, a combination of 800 IU (20 µg, or micrograms) vitamin D and 1.2 grams elemental calcium per day increased bone density in the upper leg by 2.7 percent compared with a decrease of 4.6 percent in those taking the placebo.[41] In this study, fractures were also markedly reduced. The general consensus now is that calcium and vitamin D can lower bone mineral density loss moderately and fracture rates significantly in both men and women.

Vitamin D is converted and broken down in the body into different forms (analogues and metabolites). These metabolites function to help calcium absorption and prevent loss via the kidneys, but in certain circumstances one also removes calcium from the bones. For this reason and others, it is quite possible to overdose on this vitamin; therefore, you should not exceed the label dosage.

An increase in vitamin D concentrations (achieved by thirty minutes of sunlight exposure to the face, arms, and lower legs) is associated with 5 to 10 percent increase in bone density, and such an increase may result in a 20 percent decrease in fractures.[42] Although excess sunlight is harmful to the skin, especially in fair-skinned people living in hot climates, a

TABLE 8.3 **Foods Rich in Vitamin D**

Food	Vitamin D (IU/100 g)
Sardines, canned	500
Tuna, canned	400
Salmon, canned	350
Shrimp	150
Butter	90
Eggs	50
Mushrooms	40
Natural cheese	30
Liver	30
Cream	17
Beef steak	13
Whole milk	4

I IU = 0.025 µg (micrograms).

Note: Due to natural variability these figures are approximate.

little early morning and late afternoon sun is very beneficial for the mind, body, and bones.

The calcium supplement I commonly prescribe for osteoporosis contains 100 IU (2.5 µg) of vitamin D_3 (cholecalciferol), and the daily dose is two tablets. If you are living in a cold climate, however, you may benefit from a higher dose, but unless advised otherwise by your practitioner, never take more than 800 IU (20 µg) daily.

Vitamin D supplementation in conjunction with HRT may produce harmful lipid metabolism.

CALCIUM

It's a fact that our bones become weaker as we age, especially after menopause. Calcium is a primary part of bone structure, and a deficiency of this mineral is a cause of osteoporosis. When the body levels of calcium are low, levels of the body's calcitriol increase (in an effort to increase calcium absorption). This increase stimulates the release of parathyroid hormone, which in turn stimulates the breakdown of bone cells.

For every study showing that lifelong calcium intake is linked to bone density or fracture rates, there seems to be a study showing no association.[43] The problem with population studies is that they tend to look at one or a few factors when many different factors may be affecting calcium metabolism. Some studies of even large doses of supplemental calcium have not always been successful because of other factors.

In women with osteoporosis the aim is to provide a calcium supplement that will be optimally absorbed but that will not interfere with other nutrients. For example, vitamin D is necessary for the uptake of calcium, which is why these two nutrients are often prescribed together for osteoporosis patients. One study on 3,270 elderly women showed that 1.2 grams of elemental calcium and 800 IU (20 µg) of vitamin D_3 daily for eighteen months gave a significant increase in bone mineral density and reduced fractures.[44]

Calcium supplements can prevent the 2 percent loss of bone mineral density that occurs with aging in up to half the women who take it.[45] Thus, calcium helps prevent bone loss in only 50 percent of women.

Very high doses of calcium supplementation are not recommended because it can reduce the uptake of other essential minerals and trace elements and may cause unwanted calcification in the body. Also, a number of postmenopausal women complain that high-dose calcium exacerbates arthritic symptoms and causes gastric upsets. Very high doses of calcium tend to encourage inefficient rather than thrifty metabolism.

Estrogen therapy increases the risk of clots; therefore, estrogen therapy in conjunction with high calcium and low magnesium may further increase the risk of clots. Women on HRT who take calcium supplementation make better bone improvements than women on HRT alone.[46]

Yet, there are positive side effects of calcium.

- Calcium supplements may help lower high blood pressure in people with low dietary calcium intakes.
- Dietary supplementation with calcium may help prevent the development of colorectal cancer.
- Calcium is necessary for nerve and muscle functioning.

Dietary Calcium

Countries whose populations have a high consumption of dairy foods tend to show a high incidence of osteoporosis. These same countries have diets high in protein, salt, fat, sugar, and alcohol, and the level of physical activity is generally low.

An analysis of over a hundred plant foods used by recent hunter-gatherers supports the notion that high levels of dietary calcium intake are desirable.[47] Wild vegetable foods average about 130 milligrams of calcium per 100 gram portion, which is considerably higher than modern vegetables. Plant foods would have given Stone Age people about 1,800 milligrams of calcium daily, the meat they ate would have given them another 100 milligrams, and chewing bones from birds or small mammals might have substantially increased this intake. Stone Age adults had large, strong bones, but they didn't consume dairy foods.

How Much Calcium Do We Get from Our Foods?

No one has to rely solely or mainly on dairy products to get an adequate calcium intake. (See Table 8.4.) Although the dairy industry promotes the consumption of dairy foods with each meal, that may not be in the best interests of health. For example, the addition of milk, milkshakes, or cheese to common meals such as pizza or hamburger reduces iron absorption by 50 to 60 percent. Remember also that the higher the protein intake the higher the level of calcium excretion.

TABLE 8.4 Calcium-Rich Foods

Food	Calcium (mg/100 g)	How to Use
Sesame seeds (whole raw)	1,160	Sesame seeds are best when ground to a paste; they are almost impossible to chew. They are a good source of phytoestrogens but are very high in calories. Tahini is ground sesame seeds and is used as a butter substitute.
Kelp	1,093	Amounts of kelp used are generally small, so it is not a valuable source of calcium. Also, get assurance from the supplier that the kelp is not contaminated. Some other types of edible seaweed could be used in the diet, perhaps a few times weekly; they are a rich source not only of calcium but of potassium, iodine, other nutrients, and anticancer compounds and they help digestion.
Swiss cheese (natural)	950	Many cheeses are excellent sources of calcium, although the high salt and fat content probably reduce calcium uptake. Milk is a common allergen, and a proportion of the aging population is sensitive or intolerant to all dairy foods. I use cheese more as a flavoring agent.
Whole-milk dairy powder	900	
Cheddar cheese (natural)	860	

(continued overleaf)

TABLE 8.4 *(continued)*

Food	Calcium (mg/100g)	How to Use
Whey powder (dry)	646	Whey powder is derived from cow's milk but does not have the same degree of sensitivity reactions as dairy foods. Major advantages are that it contains compounds that help balance bacteria in the digestive tract and that it improves nutrient absorption. I recommend 10 to 20 grams daily, which can be used in drinks or mixed into foods.
Sardines (canned in oil)	358	Canned salmon is another good source of calcium if the bones are retained; you can soften the bones by squeezing vinegar or lemon juice over them before serving. Salmon is highly recommended because it is are also rich in vitamin D.
Carob powder	352	How much carob powder can you eat? Using it liberally in cookies is the best way of getting a reasonable quantity. Many carob products contain a high level of sugar and additives. Read the labels.
Soy milk (dry)	330	Soy milk is commonly broken down with water but can be used, for example, in biscuits and rice desserts. It is a good source of menopausal phytoestrogens. Some people, however, are allergic to soy.

TABLE 8.4 *(continued)*

Food	Calcium (mg/100 g)	How to Use
Chocolate (plain milk)	295	Chocolate is not a recommended calcium supplement because of the high sugar content.
Linseed or flaxseed (whole raw)	271	Linseed or flaxseed is best ground to a meal and added to porridge, cereals, cookies, meat loaf, and so on. It has the added advantages of being beneficial to the digestive tract and being a good source of menopausal phytoestrogens.
Parsley (raw)	260	How much parsley can you eat? I suggest a maximum of a handful daily; it is worth using regularly because it contains menopausal phytoestrogens.
Soy grits	252	Soy grits are tastier and quicker to cook than soybeans. They can be cooked in many dishes, including porridge, rice dishes, and nut- or meat loaves. They also contain menopausal phytoestrogens.
Collard	250	The young leaves of collard, a green vegetable, may be used in salads or lightly steamed. It is not commonly available but is very easy to grow in a cool climate. Most green vegetables are reasonable sources of calcium and are highly recommended for their nutrients and anticancer compounds.

(continued overleaf)

TABLE 8.4 (*continued*)

Food	Calcium (mg/100 g)	How to Use
Almond kernels (natural raw)	245	Most nuts and seeds are good sources of calcium, but all are high in calories. I try to have a few table-spoons of them every second day.
Figs (dried)	240	
Soybeans	226	
Watercress (raw)	192	
Dandelion greens	187	
Brazil nuts	186	
(low fat)	163	

Foods such as chickpeas, yogurt, beans, onions, eggs, broccoli, spinach, buckwheat, soy milk, and wheat bran contain between 100 to 150 mg of calcium per 100 g. Most foods contain some calcium; for example, an orange has 54 mg, and a cup of mixed vegetables has about 50 mg.

Other foods such as yeast and molasses are quite high in calcium, but they have disadvantages. Yeast is used in only very small quantities and commonly causes digestive upsets; molasses has a high sugar content, contains pesticide residues, and in some countries is not recommended for human consumption.

Note: These figures are approximate because there are natural variations in the nutrient levels of all foods.

CALCIUM-RICH COOKIES

This useful recipe makes about thirty to thirty-five small cookies, each of which contains about 100 milligrams of calcium if the ingredients are used exactly as given below. These cookies are somewhat chewy; you can add more or less of the dry ingredients according to your taste. (This recipe is not low calorie.)

5 tablespoons honey
5 tablespoons tahini
1 cup mixed dried fruit
1 cup almond meal (or crushed nuts)
1 cup flaxseed meal
1 cup whey powder
½ cup carob powder
½ cup buckwheat kernels
½ cup millet meal (or oatmeal)
½ cup soy milk powder or skim milk powder
½ cup dried coconut (optional)

Melt honey and tahini in a large saucepan (don't boil). (Tahini is crushed sesame seeds, which I use as a butter substitute.)

Add the remaining ingredients to the saucepan and mix thoroughly.

Tip the mixture into a large greased baking dish and flatten with your hands. (Run your hands under cold water so that the mix doesn't stick to your fingers.)

Bake in a low oven (150°C/340°F) for about thirty minutes.

When still slightly warm, cut into small squares.

Store in the refrigerator.

An optional extra is to melt a large carob block in a little oil over low heat, add a teaspoon of vanilla extract and pour over the cookies while they are hot.

Calcium Supplements

Due to the high-protein, relatively low-calcium dietary intake of Western diets, many women benefit from calcium supplementation. Supplements are sold in different types and strengths. Table 8.5 lists the elemental calcium in some common supplements. If you buy, for example, 1,000 milligrams tablets of calcium carbonate, the actual quantity of calcium (known as elemental calcium) is 400 milligrams per tablet. It is not a false labeling because calcium has to be bound to something else for it to be absorbed.

TABLE 8.5 **Elemental Calcium in Some Common Supplements**

Supplement	Percent of Calcium	Supplement	Percent of Calcium
Calcium carbonate[a]	40	Calcium ascorbate[b]	11
Microcrystalline hydroxyapatite	24	Calcium gluconate	9
Calcium citrate	22	Bone meal (calcium	33
Calcium chelate	20	phosphate)[c]	
Calcium lactate	18	Oyster shell[c]	37
Calcium orotate	12	Dolomite[c]	20

[a]Probably poorly absorbed in older people.
[b]Primarily a vitamin C supplement.
[c]May be contaminated with heavy metals such as lead.
Note: I do not recommend bone meal, oyster shell, and dolomite; they are often contaminated, not well absorbed, and not properly evaluated. Also, calcium orotate, ascorbate, and gluconate contain too little calcium to justify their use as calcium supplements.

The calcium in acetate, lactate, gluconate, citrate, and carbonate and in whole milk is generally absorbed at somewhere between 24 to 41 percent. Some researchers, however, put calcium carbonate absorption rate as low as 3 percent, dietary calcium at around 30 percent, and calcium orotate at up to 80 percent.

I currently prescribe only two types of calcium: microcrystalline hydroxyapatite and a complex containing calcium citrate.

Microcrystalline Hydroxyapatite The product I use contains 300 milligrams elemental calcium per tablet. My standard dosage is one tablet before breakfast and one before bed. The evening tablet is taken with a little soy milk or cow's milk. This dosage interferes less with iron and other nutrients and should effectively be absorbed. Because most calcium is lost from the bones during rest, it seems reasonable that half the dosage should be taken last thing at night.

Advantages of microcrystalline hydroxyapatite include the following:

- It has been shown to restore bone.
- It may reduce pain associated with osteoporosis.
- It can accelerate the pattern and quality of bone healing.[48]
- It contains the structural component of bone as well as trace minerals needed for growth and repair of bone. The ratio of calcium, magnesium, and phosphorus is the same as that found in human bones. (If you simply grind down animal bone, it is not absorbable.)

Disadvantages include the following:

- Because it is derived from the bones of cows, hydroxyapatite could contain relatively high quantities of lead, aluminum, mercury, arsenic, and strontium. Animal and human bones accumulate and store these toxic compounds. The manufacturers I buy from have assured me that their product comes from young calves and that testing shows the products to be perfectly safe. (These heavy metals are industrial or naturally occurring in the soil, plants, and water, and the body can handle tiny amounts. Check with your manufacturer if you are concerned about the level of toxins.)
- A few people have complained that this supplement has aggravated arthritis or caused nausea. If that happens to you, check that you are not overdosing or start with a lower dose and gradually build up. If still unsuccessful, consult a health practitioner or switch to calcium citrate.

Calcium Citrate   The product I currently prescribe contains 250 milligrams of elemental calcium plus 2.5 micrograms of vitamin D_3; 125 milligrams elemental magnesium; and a small quantity of silicon, manganese, and zinc.

The dosage is one tablet before breakfast and one tablet before bed. The evening tablet is taken with a little soy milk or cow's milk.

Advantages of calcium citrate include the following:

- Calcium citrate is better absorbed than calcium carbonate.
- At a dose of between 500 to 1,500 milligrams a day, calcium citrate is more effective than calcium carbonate in osteoporotic patients. It

can reduce bone loss in postmenopausal women with a low dietary calcium intake.

- The addition of trace minerals and vitamin D improves the effect of calcium citrate malate on bone density and reduces fracture risk.[49]
- It may be the most appropriate calcium supplement for people with low stomach acid; for those with arthritis where calcification is known or suspected, or where there is unhealthy calcification in the body.
- Citrate is a good carrier of calcium. It keeps calcium in solution, mops up heavy metals, acts as a mild diuretic, and may help prevent urinary tract infections (although it is thought that very high doses of calcium carbonate may increase the risk of urinary tract infections).
- I have not observed any side effects in my clinic, and it is currently my preferred calcium supplement.

Disadvantages include the following:

- The elemental calcium content is only 22 percent, so you have to swallow a very large tablet to get a therapeutic dose.
- It is somewhat more expensive than calcium carbonate.

Rather than use very high dose calcium, I recommend a healthy diet, as outlined throughout this book, plus other supplements as indicated in appendix IV. In other words, you should be getting most nutrients from your foods. I am not relying on calcium alone to help improve bone health because if your diet is deficient in calcium, it is likely to be deficient in other nutrients. Also, osteoporosis is a serious problem; it is difficult to treat, and there are a number of possible causes.

When to Take Calcium Supplements

After menopause, the rate of overnight calcium loss in the urine increases, which is why most researchers suggest taking calcium supplements before bed. When you're sleeping, your bones and muscles are not active, so during this relatively short period of inactivity, you lose additional bone calcium similar to that which occurs during prolonged bed rest. I recommend the following guidelines for taking calcium supplements:

- Divided doses give much greater absorption than one single dose.
- Take half the dose of all supplements for osteoporosis before breakfast and half before bed.
- Many women tolerate the nighttime dose better than the morning dose, and the bone results are more effective if the supplements are taken with a protein drink. I now recommend swallowing them with about ½ cup soy milk or cow's milk.
- For supplements to be effective for osteoporosis treatment and prevention, they need to be adequate in dosage, absorbable, and taken consistently over a period of at least one year.

How to Make Your Own Calcium Supplements

EGGSHELL AND VINEGAR

Soak one finely crushed eggshell in two teaspoons or one dessert spoon of apple cider vinegar.
Let stand in a jar for twenty-four hours.
Strain and use the vinegar on food or with juice.

You will notice that the vinegar does not taste acidic any more because it has extracted the calcium out of the shell. Vinegar is a weak acetic acid, and the calcium in the vinegar (calcium acetate) should be relatively well absorbed in the body.

I had a laboratory test the vinegar, and it showed that the two teaspoons had 376 milligrams of elemental calcium in it. Generally, that amount would be a suitable daily supplement for people on a preventive program. The disadvantage is that the level of calcium will vary according to the size and quality of the eggshells. Also, shells (like bones) accumulate toxins, so if you use this method, you should buy organic eggs.

Stock Made from Bones   When making soup stock or soup from bones, add about I teaspoon of apple cider vinegar for each pint of water. (Get your butcher to cut the bones.) The vinegar will dissolve some of the calcium out of the bones. You could either have a cup of the stock daily, flavored with a teaspoon of miso, or a serving of the soup made from the stock. This stock will give you extra calcium for a preventive program, although the level of calcium is somewhat uncertain. As mentioned earlier in this chapter, the problem with animal bones is that they progressively accumulate toxic metals such as aluminum and lead. Therefore, it would be wise to use bones only from young animals for this purpose.

You should not attempt to simply grind down eggshells or bones because they are not absorbable and may irritate your digestive tract.

Calcium Toxicity

I could not find a definitive statement regarding toxic levels of calcium, but a May 14, 1986, article in the *New Zealand Medical Journal* warned about over-the-counter antacids because kidney damage has been shown to occur at levels of between 4,000 and 8,000 milligrams a day of calcium. Some antacid tablets contain 750 milligrams of calcium carbonate, and some people tend to chew them like candy. It has been suggested that these types of products should contain a warning to the effect that more than 2,000 milligrams of calcium a day may be harmful. Some antacids also contain aluminum, which is not only generally toxic and but also harmful to bones.

Excess calcium can cause a potentially life-threatening condition known as *hypercalcemia*, or milk-alkali syndrome. Always read the labels of all supplements and drugs carefully, and never exceed the dosage unless so prescribed by your health practitioner.

Antibiotics, such as tetracyclines, affect calcium so that both the calcium and the antibiotics become unabsorbable. If you are on pharmaceuticals, you should discuss any supplementation with your health practitioner because of possible interactions.

OTHER NUTRIENTS LINKED TO BONE HEALTH

Protein

I rarely prescribe a protein supplement, although I recommend that some vegetarian and elderly osteoporotic patients need to increase their protein intake by adding two servings of lean meat a week plus two or more servings of fish. A vegetarian option is to use food combining to ensure eating a complete protein, such as having a grain plus a legume in one meal for optimal protein utilization. Details of food combining are given in Frances Moore Lappé's excellent book *Diet for a Small Planet.*

Excess animal protein, however, may actually promote osteoporosis by increasing calcium excretion.[50] In all developed countries, major dietary surveys indicate that the majority of people are consuming more than twice the World Health Organization's recommended intake of protein—which is 45 grams a day for a menopausal woman. The exceptions are some categories of vegetarians, extreme dieters, the frail and elderly, those with serious chronic diseases, and those living in poverty.

Nutrients and Remedies That Help Bone Collagen (Matrix)

The bone structure or framework is mostly protein, which explains why bones need adequate but not excessive protein intake. Studies have showed that copper, manganese, and zinc supplementation help osteoporosis. Each of these studies demonstrated the necessity of trace elements for optimal bone matrix development and bone density sustenance.[51]

Aside from amino acids—including proline, glutamine, lysine, and cystine—other nutrients thought to help collagen metabolism are silica, magnesium, manganese, iron, vitamin B_5, vitamin B_6, and vitamin C.

Various remedies purported to help collagen can be considered. They include glucosamine, chondroitin sulfate, green-lipped mussels, flavonoids, liquid bovine tracheal cartilage, shark cartilage, and gotu kola. These compounds and herbs are also in natural therapies' arthritis remedies.

Bone is more than a collection of calcium crystals. Active living bone cells need a wide range of nutrients and a healthy blood supply, with a balance between bone breakdown and bone building.[52] Nutrients work as a team. Any nutrient in excess will either interfere with other nutrients or cause side effects. Good nutrition must also be supported by physical activity and a healthy lifestyle.

Finally, osteoporosis is a serious and complicated problem. My experience may not necessarily be relevant to your particular case, and you should always discuss treatment with a practitioner who can guide and monitor your progress.

CHAPTER NINE

Health After Menopause

*A*fter you have maneuvered your way through menopause and you're confident that your bones are in adequate condition, it's time to look at the problems that occur as you age and to do all that is reasonable to prevent premature aging.

The basic recommendations for menopause and osteoporosis still apply after menopause. The one exception is that you can cut back somewhat on the quantity of phytoestrogens you eat now that your hot flashes have passed.

A varied whole-food diet is necessary for good health at any age for a number of reasons.

- It provides the most nutrients, some of which are not on current government essential nutrient lists. Government recommended intakes for most nutrients are conservative and are based on quantities that will prevent deficiency diseases rather than on quantities that will provide optimal health and lifespan. Some trace elements, flavonoids, and other compounds are not yet classified as essential.
- Foods in their natural state provide hundreds of phytochemicals, such as antioxidants, that have disease-preventing properties.

- All plants contain toxins that are needed by the plant itself. If you eat a variety of foods, it is unlikely that you will get a buildup of a particular toxin. (A healthy body has a mechanism for dealing with the tiny amounts of naturally occurring toxins in edible and medicinal plants.)
- Manufactured and processed foods contain manufactured chemicals. It is unknown how all these interact with each other.

Every major dietary survey carried out in the United States indicates that a significant proportion of elderly people are consuming a diet that falls far short of the basic recommended intakes of many nutrients, even though these recommended intakes are relatively low and do not include all the trace elements and antioxidants that many researchers now consider vital for health.

The word *supplement* actually means "something added to supply deficiencies, especially fuller treatment or addition." Many people will benefit from appropriate supplementation because most of our food is not freshly harvested and contains added chemicals, but a supplement is not a substitute for healthy food. In the absence of practitioner advice, always observe the label dosages of foods and supplements. Exercise and a health-enhancing (but nonfanatical) lifestyle and philosophy are equally necessary.

As discussed in chapter 2, HRT is currently being promoted as being protective against heart disease, stroke, and dementia, although these claims are questionable. In any event, it does not seem reasonable to recommend HRT for prevention when the therapy itself carries with it a long list of potentially harmful effects.

It is not possible to cover all the problems of aging in one chapter, so I focus on healthy preventive options that may be helpful for the major problems: heart and circulatory diseases, stroke, and dementia as well as some aspects of cancer prevention. This chapter provides a brief overview of some relevant preventive and early treatment strategies.

HEART DISEASE

Your heart and blood vessels have a major effect on how you age and how you feel, and heart disease is the main cause of death in all developed countries.

Symptoms of heart and circulatory problems include chest, neck, and arm pain; breathlessness from minimal activity; headaches; numbness in the fingers, and palpitations or other heartbeat irregularities, which should all be medically checked. Have your blood pressure and cholesterol levels monitored periodically because high levels can cause damage if not corrected. If discovered in the early stages, cholesterol levels and high blood pressure can be treated successfully with natural remedies as long as you are also willing to make dietary and lifestyle changes.

Basic Dietary Preventive Measures

There is considerable evidence that specific types of diets lower the risk of heart and circulatory disorders. Basic recommendations are as follows:

1. Eat at least five servings of fresh fruit and vegetables each day. Fruit and vegetables are the best foods to provide a wide range of antioxidants and antiaging compounds. Five servings are not excessive if you have, for example, a piece of fruit with breakfast, a salad or soup with lunch, a piece of fruit for an afternoon snack or before dinner, and cooked vegetables as part of your evening meal. Well over a hundred studies support the role of antioxidants for preventing heart disease, and fruit and vegetables are the best source of antioxidants.

2. Significantly reduce animal products. Unless you have an allergy or sensitivity problem, include some low-fat yogurt, low-fat milk, and small quantities of lean meats in your diet. Eggs, which are rich in protein and other essential nutrients, are suggested four times per week. They are relatively high in fats but tend to increase HDL (high density lipoprotein), the "good" cholesterol.

   Excess iron may lead to excess oxidation in the body, which is why a low-meat diet is suggested and why you should avoid iron supplements unless your physician has diagnosed anemia. One way of offsetting excess iron is to donate blood.[1] The good news is that male blood donors were shown to have an 88 percent reduced risk of acute heart attacks compared with men who did not give blood. Other potential problems of a high meat diet are covered in chapters 6 and 8.

3. Increase plant protein. Recommended foods include whole brown rice, lentils, soybeans and soy products, chickpeas, beans, and all whole grains and legumes. Whole grains and legumes are rich in nutrients and antioxidants and have other cardiovascular benefits. Also, use small quantities of nuts and seeds (except peanuts, which often contain aflatoxins, naturally occurring liver toxins). Combining a legume with a grain or nuts and seeds or with dairy products provides more effective protein utilization.

   The Nurses Health Study, which followed 84,409 American nurses for fourteen years to examine the link between diet and heart disease, found that women who ate more than 5 ounces (and/or 150 grams) of nuts per week had a 35 percent lower risk of coronary heart disease than women who never ate nuts or who ate less than 1 ounce per month.[2] Try not to eat too many nuts and seeds, however, because they are high in calories.

   This group of foods can also be used as meat extenders. For example, cooked lentils can be included in a meat loaf and soy flakes can be used to thicken a casserole.

4. Fish is highly recommended. The types of fish that contain the most beneficial "heart oils" include cold water fish like salmon, sardines, mackerel, trout, and eel.

   It's quite difficult to be a healthy vegetarian, so for most people I suggest consuming some animal products as well as fish.

5. Reduce salt intake. For flavoring, use a little low-sodium tamari (soy sauce), lemon, vinegar, and culinary herbs.

6. Reduce the intake of animal fat and refined sugars. Use these foods as treats and develop the habit of filling up on health-enhancing foods.

7. Reduce processed foods in your diet. Processed foods contain fewer nutrients and more synthetic chemicals than foods in a natural state.

Some Specific Heart Foods

Olive Oil   The Mediterranean diet includes olive oil, garlic, fresh fruit, vegetables, and red wine and has less red meat than typical British and American diets. Extra virgin olive oil contains a number of beneficial oils plus compounds such as polyphenols, which are powerful antioxidants. Generally, Mediterraneans have a high level of dietary antioxidants if they stick to their traditional diet. The benefits of traditional cold-pressed olive oil are largely lost when the oils are manufactured using heat, solvents, hydrogenation, and other processes that alter the chemistry.

Black Grapes   Although Mediterraneans have a lower incidence of heart disease compared with other Europeans, the French have a three-fold higher death rate from lung cancer, cirrhosis, and alcoholism compared with British people. Too much wine is not healthy. I have lived in and visited many different countries and France is the only country where people respond to a simple "How are you" with "J'ai mal au foie" ("My liver's bad").

One glass of red wine for women and two glasses for men is probably the daily level that will provide some benefits without adverse effects (except for people with liver diseases, who should have no alcohol whatsoever). I'm sure that black grapes are healthier than wine, but they are not as relaxing and enjoyable!

Tea   A study of tea and coffee drinkers found that those who drank one or more cups of tea daily had about half the risk of heart attacks compared with those who drank no tea.[3] Drink at least two cups of weak black or green tea per day, perhaps with a slice of lemon or some grated ginger for flavoring. If you add milk, the beneficial tannins cannot be absorbed, which cuts out the valuable antioxidant effect.

Garlic and Fiber-rich Foods: Whole Grains, Vegetables, Fruit, Legumes
Garlic, herbs, and many plant foods are good sources of antioxidants and have many other health benefits.

Remedies That Help the Heart

Many individual antioxidants and other supplements may reduce the risk of heart disease. It has been shown that vitamins C and E, glutathione, and coenzyme Q10 offer more antioxidant protection than a single supplement. There is, however, a wider variety of antioxidants in foods and herbs than in any pill.

Vitamin E   There are hundreds of scientific papers supporting the benefits of vitamin E for the heart and circulation, and it should be the number one supplement for all people over fifty.

Coenzyme Q10   A scientific trial of seventy-three people who had suffered heart attacks showed that 120 milligrams a day of coenzyme Q10 reduced angina, irregular heartbeat, and ventricular function compared with those on placebo.[4] This dosage of coenzyme Q10 also reduces blood pressure in most people.

Lecithin   Lecithin contains a number of useful substances, including choline (a B vitamin). Choline has many functions in the body and reduces the levels of excess homocysteine, a damaging amino acid. Four months on soybean lecithin lowered total blood lipids, cholesterol, and triglycerides in patients with high levels.[5] Lecithin is also helpful for brain and liver functioning.

B Vitamins   High levels of homocysteine are linked to a higher incidence of cardiovascular and other diseases related to aging, including osteoporosis. When folate (vitamin B_9)and vitamin B_{12} were given as supplements, homocysteine levels dropped between 25 to 33 percent, according to a summary of twelve trials.[6] The combination of cigarette smoking and high coffee intake is associated with particularly high homocysteine concentrations.[7] Cigarette smoking and high coffee intakes are also linked to osteoporosis. Vitamin B_6 and other vitamins have been linked to a reduction in heart disease.[8]

Magnesium   A large survey of over 13,922 men and women found that low serum magnesium may contribute to the progression of coronary heart disease, especially in women.[9] Magnesium is now recommended for osteoporosis (see chapter 8.)

Fish Oil   Fish oil is also highly recommended. It also helps calcium metabolism.

Herbs That Help the Heart and Blood Vessels

Most herbs that have been used traditionally for heart problems are antioxidants and circulatory tonics and are rich in flavonoids.

Coleus   *Coleus forskohlii* has been used in India and tested in Germany and elsewhere mainly for its effect in lowering blood pressure and relaxing blood vessel walls. It should not be used if you are taking any other pharmaceuticals, however.

Garlic and Ginger   Garlic and ginger help keep the blood flow healthy. They are antioxidants and have many other benefits. Use them generously and regularly in your diet.

Hawthorn   Hawthorn is well documented for its ability to relax blood vessels and to increase blood flow and oxygen supply to the heart. It has antioxidant properties, and it can lower blood pressure and relieve angina.[10]

Terminalia   When Indian patients with heart disease due to inadequate blood flow were given 500 milligrams of the herb *Terminalia arjuna* three times daily, the flow of blood through the congested left ventricle improved compared with those who were on conventional medical treatment only.[11] The use of this herb should be practitioner supervised, but you can use ginger, garlic, and ginkgo for preventive purposes to improve circulation.

Ginkgo   Ginkgo is an antioxidant and is helpful for improving circulation and memory.[12]

Exercise

A regular, appropriate exercise pattern needs to be established so that it becomes part of your life. Exercise is a major factor in preventing heart and blood vessel problems. Chapter 7 covers exercise in some detail. Of course, if you have a heart problem, you need professional help in developing an appropriate program.

Atherosclerosis (Clogged Arteries)

Diet   Diets rich in beta-carotene are linked to a decrease in arterial plaque formation (clogged arteries).[13] Foods rich in beta-carotene include yellow and green vegetables.

Berries are recommended because they are powerful antioxidants, and components in grapes are known to reduce free radicals and cardiovascular risk factors.[14] Components in grapes are also considered to be antithrombotic and anticancer. You don't have to drink wine to get the benefits; you can eat fresh grapes, grape juice, and even raisins. All the purple-colored edible foods are highly recommended.

Numerous published studies indicate that a diet rich in fruit and vegetables protects the arteries through antioxidant effects, improving blood flow and strengthening artery walls. Isoflavonic phytoestrogens, as listed in chapters 3 and 4, improve the elasticity of blood vessel walls, have antioxidant activity, and may even help your bones.

One study showed that skipping breakfast increased the degree of platelet stickiness and the tendency for clotting. Because the risk of heart attack is the greatest early in the morning when the blood is stickier, skipping breakfast may extend the high risk hours. Wholesome food and regular eating patterns are recommended if you want to keep your blood flowing to your heart. As discussed in chapter 6, excess dieting (which includes missing meals) is not good for bone health either. After fasting overnight, your brain needs a good blood flow so that it is not deprived of oxygen and nutrients. You don't need a large breakfast, just a small serving of cereal or yogurt and a piece of fruit, and perhaps a whole grain muffin midmorning.

Supplements   Vitamin E reduces the oxidation of the bad cholesterol (LDL), which is a trigger for the buildup of fatty streaks in the blood vessel walls.[15] Vitamin E also reduces blood stickiness and inflammation and helps the linings of blood vessels, which are all linked to clogged arteries. An analysis of the Cambridge Heart Antioxidant Study trial concluded "that vitamin E therapy in patients with angiographically proven atherosclerosis is cost-effective."[16] All postmenopausal women would benefit from a supplement of between 250 to 500 IU (150 to 350 mg) of vitamin E daily.[17]

Supplementation with pyridoxine, folate, and vitamin B[12] halted the progression of clogged arteries in patients over sixty-five years of age.[18] This finding is added evidence that older people can improve not only their bones but also their cardiovascular health. If three vitamins can make this difference, think what major dietary and lifestyle improvements could do.

Lifestyle   Inflammation caused by bacteria is another trigger leading to blocked arteries. Flavonoids help offset this inflammation and support the traditional use of a diet rich in citrus and other fruit, especially when you have infections. Preventing and treating infections rather than letting them linger is another useful strategy.

If you have high levels of cholesterol oxidation compounds (from LDL or VLDL, the "bad" forms of cholesterol), you are more likely to get atherosclerosis (clogged arteries). Harmful oxidation compounds are also linked to cigarette smoking.[19]

Your artery walls include bands of smooth muscles, and regular exercise helps keep them flexible. A group of researchers found some evidence that doing work under time pressure correlates with platelet aggregation (blood clumping) and suggest that such clumping may provide an explanation of the link between hostility and anger (type-A personality) and coronary heart disease.[20] Various mind-body practices—such as social support, counseling, behavioral therapy, medication, faith, imagery, spiritual healing, music therapy, hypnosis, tai chi, yoga, and qi gong[21]—can provide complementary treatment for heart-related conditions.

HIGH CHOLESTEROL

Foods That Help Lower the Bad Cholesterol (LDL and VLDL)

At least one medical study confirms that each of the following foods can lower harmful cholesterol if the levels are high, so include them in your diet on a regular basis. If your blood cholesterol is not high, eat the above foods anyway because they have many other benefits.

- Soybeans
- Whole grains
- Alfalfa
- Fish
- Wheat germ
- Pectin (as in apples)
- Flaxseed meal
- Citrus fiber (that is, the whole fruit, not juices)
- Oyster mushrooms
- Maitake, reishi, and other medicinal mushrooms
- Blueberries and blackberries
- Almonds, hazelnuts, and walnuts
- Sunflower seeds
- Extra virgin olive oil
- Oat, barley, and rice bran
- Vegetables and legumes
- Whey protein (as in whey powder)
- Buckwheat
- Rhubarb stalk
- Psyllium
- Lecithin
- Lactobacillus

A number of trials indicate that soybeans and soy products that contain the protein and fiber of soy are helpful for lowering cholesterol.[22] The isoflavones in soybeans and soy products also act as antioxidants to protect against the harmful breakdown of LDL cholesterol.[23] Linseeds have similar antioxidant effects.

Cholesterol-Lowering Supplements

The following supplements are known to reduce cholesterol levels:
- Niacin
- Vitamin C
- Fructooligosaccharides
- Grapeseed extract
- Chitosan

Cholesterol-Lowering Herbs

Some cholesterol-lowering herbs can be added into your normal diet. Ginger and turmeric, for example, are excellent antioxidants, and they both aid digestion and circulation. Anything that aids your digestion and circulation will also benefit your bones, heart, and brain. Cholesterol-lowering herbs include the following:

- Garlic
- Milk thistle (*Silybum*)
- Turmeric
- Ginger
- Bilberry
- Chili peppers
- Cat's claw
- Hawthorn

At least thirteen scientific studies have demonstrated that garlic is effective at lowering both total and LDL cholesterol. My clinical experience is that the best results are obtained if concentrated, powdered enteric-coated garlic capsules are used; these capsules do not cause odor and reflux problems, and each capsule provides the equivalent of about 5 grams of garlic. Two to four capsules daily, together with a liver remedy and dietary modifications, usually produce a reduction of about 15 percent in two months. After that, a cholesterol maintenance program is generally sufficient.

My observation is that when total cholesterol is reduced, the bad cholesterol is proportionately reduced. High cholesterol is usually caused because the liver produces too much; hence, my treatment includes a liver remedy such as guaranteed potency milk thistle that gives between 300 to 400 milligrams of silymarin daily for two months, followed by a lower maintenance dose.

Overemphasis on low cholesterol levels is a problem because some people without heart problems are fooled into thinking that an extremely low level is healthier. Cholesterol has many necessary functions in the body, including the production of sex hormones. Low cholesterol is also linked to violence and suicide. A reason may be lowered serotonin, a neurotransmitter that modifies behavior. Therefore, people with low cholesterol may be more likely to respond inappropriately to adverse life circumstances.[24] Very low cholesterol is also associated with a lowered antioxidant status; thin people, who are obsessed with physical fitness and low-fat foods, may be more at risk because prolonged and excessive activity also increases oxidation products.

A few studies show that very elderly people with high cholesterol have less cancer and infectious diseases, but these people may be the exceptionally hardy individuals whose bodies can tolerate high animal fats and unhealthy lifestyle habits.

Lifestyle

People who practiced transcendental meditation were shown to have low lipid peroxide levels,[25] which means that the stress-reducing effects of meditation appear to lower the harmful by-products (oxidation) of fat metabolism. A study on Indian soldiers also showed that yogic breathing techniques, when practiced daily, lowered both cholesterol and glucose levels.[26] Aerobic exercise also has a beneficial effect on cholesterol.

Cholesterol-lowering drugs have many adverse effects, including liver damage. If you have a major heart problem that requires these pharmaceutical drugs, at least lower your alcohol intake and take a guaranteed potency milk thistle product to protect the liver. These pharmaceutical drugs also damage carotenoids, such as lutein, that are essential for eye health, so make sure you eat green leafy vegetables every day. It has also been suggested that coenzyme Q10 supplementation may offset some of the harmful effects of cholesterol-lowering pharmaceuticals.

What to Avoid

- Coffee, especially boiled
- Excess alcohol
- High dietary animal fats
- Sugar and sugary foods (except the sugar in whole fruit)
- Excess eggs (a few each week should not be a problem because eggs tend to increase the good cholesterol, or HDL)

HYPERTENSION

Pressure (tension) in the arteries can rise to an unsafe level due to fluid retention, kidney function, high cholesterol, atherosclerosis, hardened arterial walls, and obesity; sometimes no specific cause can be found.

Diet

The same dietary guidelines for heart disease apply to hypertension. Because vegetarians have a significantly lower incidence of hypertension, unless you have a severe problem requiring immediate pharmaceutical control, you could try a strict vegetarian diet for two months while having your blood pressure monitored regularly. A diet rich in fruit and vegetables with reduced animal fats can reduce blood pressure.[27] An appropriate weight loss program, including exercise, often lowers blood pressure.

Herbs That Help Lower Blood Pressure

A qualified herbalist can make up an individualized formula that may include some of the following herbs in accordance with your health status. Individual herbs have more than one action, so the selection might also relate to other problems that you have, such as chronic stress. One remedy alone, such as a cup of chamomile tea, is unlikely to make any difference to blood pressure, although it would be more beneficial than, for example, a cup of coffee.

- Celery
- Coleus
- Chamomile
- Fenugreek
- Hawthorn
- Linden (lime flowers)
- Garlic
- Ginkgo
- Olive leaves
- Skullcap
- Siberian ginseng (antistress)
- Yarrow

Supplements

A daily magnesium supplement can give modest reductions in high blood pressure.[28]

Exercise

I always recommend an exercise program. Many people also benefit from a stress management or meditation course.

During one trial that involved a twelve-week walking program, blood pressure readings were significantly lower in a group of postmenopausal women. For three weeks they walked for thirty minutes three to four days a week; the walking speed was then increased and the time extended to forty-five minutes.[29] Blood pressure readings decreased throughout the trial, indicating that a longer-term program would probably continue to normalize blood pressure and would also produce other benefits.

Aerobic exercise also increases DHEA, an adrenal hormone that is produced in the body and that is currently promoted in pill form as a restorative hormone. When a DHEA pill was given to postmenopausal exercisers, however, it also increased the levels of lactic acid and cortisol in those on hormone replacement therapy, suggesting a stress response. Given that excess cortisol is linked to premature aging, bone loss, immune system suppression, and connective tissue weakness, I recommend that you increase your DHEA the natural way by exercising regularly and vigorously. You may, however, need to start exercising very slowly and steadily build up because your blood vessels may not tolerate a sudden surge of activity.

Lifestyle

People who regularly practiced transcendental meditation showed a reduction of 9 mmHg diastolic blood pressure after four months.[30] A study of 942 men over four years showed that those with the highest feelings of hopelessness were more likely to have atherosclerotic thickening (narrowed arteries).[31] When the arteries are narrowed, blood pressure usually increases and blood vessels and blood flow are under stress.

Based on my clinical experience and on a few published studies, some people seem to have high blood pressure only when the doctor takes the measurement. This situation is called "white coat hypertension" and is probably a nervous response. You may want to get a second opinion, have someone else check your blood pressure, or rent the equipment so that you can check your blood pressure three times daily for a few weeks. In some cases, monitoring is a better option than taking pharmaceutical drugs because it may indicate that your blood pressure is not actually high but is occasionally reactive.

CIRCULATORY DISORDERS

To maintain your health, you need to strengthen blood vessel walls, reduce inflammation, and improve blood flow. The following various natural therapies can help.

Diet

Buckwheat, fiber-rich foods, and fruit all improve circulation. Buckwheat is rich in rutin—which helps keep blood vessel walls strong—and lowers

LDL cholesterol. Buckwheat is available in many forms, including crackers, flour, and pasta, or you can cook the kernels in various ways. It is quite bland, so it needs plenty of flavoring.

BUCKWHEAT SALAD
Serves 2 as a side salad

½ cup buckwheat
1 cup water
1 small onion, finely chopped
1 small tomato, finely chopped
1 cup mushrooms, sliced
½ cup low-fat yogurt
½ small avocado, cut into small squares
2 tablespoons cashews
1 teaspoon lemon juice
1 teaspoon low-sodium soy sauce
About ¼ cup finely chopped herbs (chives, basil, parsley, rocket)
10 lettuce leaves, washed

Simmer the onion in water for five minutes.

Add the buckwheat and simmer for a further five minutes. Let stand until cool.

Add the remaining ingredients (except the lettuce leaves), and gently mix together.

Put into a serving bowl. Arrange the lettuce leaves on a separate plate.

Spoon about a tablespoon of the salad mix onto a lettuce leaf and roll it so that it can be eaten by hand.

Herbs and Supplements for Circulatory Health

Herbs for circulatory health include the following:

- Bilberry
- Chili peppers
- Ginger

- Ginkgo
- Hawthorn
- Horse chestnut

Supplements for circulatory health include the following:

- Grapeseed extract
- Vitamin C and flavonoids

Exercise and Lifestyle

Exercise is necessary because venous blood and lymph are moved by muscle action. Aerobic activity, yoga, and tai chi are also beneficial for circulation and general health. Correct breathing and posture are recommended because the diaphragm is the body's main pump for veins and lymph vessels. Avoid tight clothes and standing still for long periods, and whenever possible, rest with your feet up or at least use a footstool.

STROKE

Stroke is the third leading cause of death and the leading cause of long-term disability in the United States. The basic cause of stroke is a blood vessel wall problem or blood flow that is too thick or viscous (sometimes caused by high VLDL, the bad cholesterol); impeded because of hypertension, inflammation, injury, or clots; or excessively thin blood so that it flows too quickly and stresses the blood vessel walls or prevents normal healing processes.

There are different types of stroke, and all require medical attention. The recommendations for heart disease and circulatory disorders generally apply to stroke prevention.

Diet

Flavonoids are also thought to protect against stroke. The best sources of flavonoids are fruits and vegetables. A U.S. study of 75,596 women found that the risk of stroke caused by restricted blood flow was 31 percent lower in women who consumed an average of 5.8 servings of fruits and vegetables per day.[32]

Supplements and Herbs

Vitamin E is helpful for preventing excess free radicals or oxidants, which are among the triggers leading to blocked arteries. For the same reason, this vitamin may be helpful for people recovering from strokes because it may reduce the injured area of the brain.[33]

In one study, a single dose of 10 grams (about 1 teaspoon) of ginger powder reduced blood stickiness (platelet aggregation), but 4 grams a day for three months did not.[34] For improved blood flow, it might be more effective to take a high dose of ginger every second or third day rather than a low dose long-term. If you are on blood-thinning medication, do not take ginger unless approved by your physician.

Lifestyle

A follow-up of hypertension patients after eighteen to twenty-two years showed that qi gong was more effective at reducing stroke than pharmaceuticals.[35] Health-enhancing lifestyle habits need to be long term, but you don't have to wait eighteen years to get the benefits!

Tests show that the blood tends to be thicker in the presence of physical and mental stressors. Sluggish blood flow is part of various triggers that lead to high blood pressure, clogged arteries, and stroke. Emotional upsets that cause a sudden rise in blood pressure may also be a cause of stroke because the pressure may rupture small blood vessels.[36]

Treating pain and illnesses rather than tolerating them and developing strategies to offset mental stressors have long-term protective effects for stroke and heart disease. Some of these strategies are discussed in chapter 10. Try natural remedies first because regular and consistent use of aspirin and other anti-inflammatory drugs is associated with diverticular disease[37] and many other side effects. Finally, a walk a day might keep the strokes away!

General Cautions If you are on pharmaceutical drugs, always discuss any additional remedies you want to take with your doctor.

If you are about to undergo or are recovering from surgery or other medical procedures, be guided by your medical specialist.

Keys for Keeping Your Heart, Brain, and Circulation Healthy

- There is no substitute for a varied, whole-food diet if you want a healthy heart, brain, and circulatory system. Regular meals are also required.
- You must establish regular exercise habits if you want to prevent premature aging.
- Vitamin E is the paramount heart and circulatory supplement.
- Atherosclerosis, high cholesterol, and hypertension—in the early stages—can be treated successfully by diet, exercise, natural remedies, and lifestyle modifications.
- If you want a relatively long and healthy life, give up cigarette smoking and excessive intake of salt, alcohol, refined and concentrated sugars, and animal fats.
- Be aware of what is going on in your body. Signs such as breathlessness, palpitations or irregular heartbeat, pain, headaches, dizziness, blurred vision, and numbness should be checked by a physician.

DEMENTIA AND ALZHEIMER'S DISEASE

Many of my patients are concerned about loss of mental function. Although there are many possible causes of dementia and Alzheimer's disease, no one can guarantee either the prevention or treatment of them in the elderly; yet, with the exception of some relatively rare diseases, there is no evidence that they are hereditary either. If you are worried about memory loss, see your practitioner; there are basic tests to check memory function.

Several factors can lead to dysfunctions in the brain and mind.

- Aging
- Anemia
- Blood sugar problems
- Boredom/lack of stimulation
- Depression
- Disordered brain biochemistry
- Drugs, social and pharmaceutical
- Environmental and ingested toxins
- Nutritional deficiencies
- Hormonal imbalances
- Food additives
- Genetic diseases such as Huntington's disease
- Infections such as candidiasis
- Weather
- Chronic stress
- Chronic pain
- Circulatory disorders
- Lack of exercise
- Insomnia
- Allergies

Some of these causes or possibilities are only indirectly linked to memory loss. Low thyroid activity causes fatigue, for example, and you know from your own experience that if you're exhausted, your mind does not function efficiently. A deficiency of iron or folic acid can also cause poor mental functioning, as can a deficiency of any of the B vitamins.

Certain people seem to be sensitive to atmospheric influences. Various parts of the world have dry winds, which are linked to symptoms called "serotonin irritation syndrome" (serotonin is a brain chemical). Other people get depressed when they get insufficient natural light and fresh air. When you are depressed, anxious, or angry, your brain and memory don't function efficiently. It is not easy or even possible to trace and eliminate the cause of problems, but it is worth trying, even if only to help you understand what is happening to you.

Brain Aids

Ginkgo biloba   When the herb ginkgo was given to Alzheimer's patients over a one-year period, they maintained or slightly improved their mental status, whereas those on placebo deteriorated.[38] Numerous studies show that ginkgo improves age-related brain and circulatory problems, and the medical trials used guaranteed potency products. Ginkgo is not a miracle cure, and in general, at least six months' treatment is required before assessing results. Ginkgo works mainly through its flavonoids, improving circulation to the brain. It can also help lower blood pressure.[39]

Coenzyme Q10   Coenzyme Q10 is a natural antioxidant that can increase energy and lower blood pressure.

Bacopa and Gotu kola (*Centella asiatica*)   Bacopa and gotu kola are traditional Indian (Ayurvedic) brain remedies. Their effectiveness has been supported in modern scientific journals.

B-Complex Vitamins   A damaging amino acid in the body called homocysteine is also high in people with Alzheimer's disease. This amino acid is known to be lowered by specific B vitamins, notably pyridoxine (B_6), folic acid (B_9), and vitamin B_{12}.

Vitamins C and E   A survey of 633 people over sixty-five years of age showed that those who had taken vitamin C and vitamin E supplements had no signs of Alzheimer's disease.[40] Another researcher has suggested that antioxidant and anti-inflammatory drugs should be helpful in treating early forms of Alzheimer's and that large doses of vitamin C and vitamin E might be beneficial.[41] A number of medical surveys suggest that vitamin E may help ward off memory problems, and one study has shown that in patients with moderately severe impairment from Alzheimer's disease, vitamin E can slow the disease progression.[42] Vitamin E in particular seems to have preventive and treatment possibilities.

Surveys indicate that past or present intake of the main vitamins and protein are related to intellectual performance in elderly people. B vitamins and antioxidants have been consistently linked with at least modest benefits in off-setting intellectual decline in the elderly, and folic acid in particular is thought to be important for the maintenance of intellectual status in the elderly.

Glutamine   Glutamine is an amino acid that is a key building block for glutathione, an important antioxidant produced in the body. This amino acid is also used to make gamma-aminobutyric acid, a chemical messenger that acts as an antidepressant. In addition, glutamine helps increase mental alertness, increases energy, and is an important nutrient for the intestinal tract.

DHA (Docosahexaenoic Acid), as in Fish Oil   DHA is an oil component in fish that is necessary for nerve tissue membranes, which are responsible for transmitting brain messages. A study on people with manic depression showed that fish oil reduced mood swings.[43] Lack of emotional control impedes normal thought processes and is also a risk factor for strokes.

Phosphatidyl Serine   Phosphatidyl serine is a new supplement derived from soy lecithin. It is said to improve memory and concentration by helping to regenerate the nerve endings, making them more pliable and increasing the levels of brain chemical receivers (neurotransmitter receptor sites). It is reported to increase relaxation and creativity by increasing alpha waves in the brain and is said to improve mood by increasing dopamine (the brain's motivation chemical). It helps some cases of insomnia and is currently promoted as a memory nutrient.[44]

Other Anti–Alzheimer's Disease Aids   Scientific investigators report that vegetables, particularly spinach, may be beneficial in retarding age-related central nervous system and mental behavioral insufficiencies. This effect may be due to the wide range of antioxidants in vegetables that help offset the decline in the body's antioxidants that occurs with aging. A combination of ginkgo, antioxidants, and medications has been proposed for early Alzheimer's disease.[45]

Mental activity helps keep the brain young. Particularly after retirement, it is important to keep the mind active, be socially involved, learn new skills, enhance creativity, or participate in volunteer work. Of course, physical activity keeps the heart pumping so that energy and nutrients can be circulated to the brain.

What to Avoid If You Want to Prevent Premature Brain Aging

- Avoid excess alcohol and coffee.
- Avoid fluoride. Use a water filter instead. Animals fed even low doses of fluoride show more aluminum in brain tissue.
- Avoid cigarette smoking.
- Avoid excess salt, excess sugar, excess fat, and junk food. Excess sugar and sugary foods are linked to faulty collagen, and the type and amount of sugars can significantly affect the health and lifespan of elderly people.[46]
- Avoid a sedentary lifestyle.
- Avoid obesity.
- Prevent illnesses such as diabetes, hypertension and high LDL cholesterol, and stroke. If you already have any one of these problems, get practitioner help to reduce their effects because these are risk factors for vascular dementia (i.e., lowered brain function due to insufficient blood flow to the brain).

CANCER

According to a 1999 World Health Organization Data Bank, the United States had the third highest female cancer death rate (when seventeen countries were compared and the figures adjusted for age). It is therefore worthwhile to look at some steps you can take to avoid cancer.

There is considerable evidence (and speculation) that more than 70 percent of cancers are linked to inappropriate nutrition, contaminated foods, exposure to synthetic chemicals, and harmful lifestyle choices such as smoking and excess alcohol. Chapter 2 provides evidence that HRT is potentially cancer causing, whereas healthful foods are potentially cancer preventive.

Diet

The U.S. National Cancer Institute has compiled a list of cancer-preventive foods [47] (in order of importance):

1. Garlic
2. Cabbage
3. Licorice (not confectionery)
4. Soybeans
5. Ginger
6. Umbelliferae family (carrots, celery, parsnips, and probably many herbs in this family such as angelica, aniseed, caraway, chervil, coriander, cumin, dill, fennel, lovage, parsley)
7. Onions
8. Tea
9. Turmeric
10. Citrus (orange, lemon, grapefruit, mandarin)
11. Whole wheat
12. Flaxseed
13. Brown rice
14. Solanaceae family (tomato, eggplant, peppers, potato)
15. Brassicaceae family (notably broccoli, brussels sprouts, cauliflower)
16. Oats
17. Mints
18. Oregano
19. Cucumber
20. Rosemary
21. Sage
22. Potato
23. Thyme
24. Chives
25. Cantaloupe
26. Basil
27. Tarragon

28. Barley
29. Berries

With the exception of licorice, which should be used in the form of pure licorice root and at quantities of less than 3 grams a day to avoid potential side effects, there is no reason you cannot add these foods and herbs into your diet on a regular basis. If you are not sure how to incorporate the culinary herbs in this list, simply add a handful of mixed fresh herbs into a meal once daily. I also use herbal vinegar and the following anticancer vinegar recipe.

HERBAL ANTICANCER VINEGAR

2 teaspoons turmeric powder
2 teaspoons ginger powder
2 teaspoons licorice powder
Contents of two green teabags
Contents of two mint teabags
A large handful of chopped fresh herbs (choose from rosemary, oregano, tarragon, sage, thyme, basil)
I pint apple cider or balsamic vinegar

Put the ingredients in a bottle.
Seal, label, and date. Store on its side for at least a few days before use.
Sprinkle 2 teaspoons per person on salads or savory meals, or use in a salad dressing.
As the vinegar is a preservative, the remedy will keep for at least six months.
If you don't have fresh herbs, you can use dried herbs but keep them to less than 20 teaspoons; they swell once they are moistened in the vinegar.

Many studies indicate that plant foods protect against breast cancer, notably vegetables, fruits, and flaxseed; the main nutrients involved include vitamin C, vitamin E, folic acid, fiber, and the carotenoids alpha-carotene, beta-carotene, lutein, and zeaxanthin.[48] Carotenoids are found mainly in green and yellow vegetables.

Over 150 studies show that people who eat a large quantity of vegetables and fruits are up to 50 percent less likely to develop cancer than those eating a small amount. A study using tomato juice, carrot juice, and spinach powder showed that these carotenoid-rich foods reduce cell damage and may help prevent the development of cancer.[49]

Some studies using beta-carotene have produced seemingly negative effects; my interpretation is that these studies have all related to synthetic forms of beta-carotene, which seem to be detrimental, especially to smokers.

Dr. J. Michnovicz of the Foundation for Preventative Oncology states that indole-3-carbinol, a component in the cabbage family, can activate enzymes in the body that help deactivate the excessive estrogen hormones that precipitate certain cancers. Pure licorice root is also considered to encourage this anticancer metabolism in breast tissue.

A recent study suggested that postmenopausal women with low levels of vitamin B_{12} have an increased incidence of breast cancer.[50] In my practice I find a number of older women who are B_{12} deficient, with the main symptom being fatigue. This deficiency is usually not dietary but an absorption problem. When in doubt, speak to your physician.

A low antioxidant intake is also linked to an increased risk of cervical lesions (uterus) and cancer.[51] Again, the emphasis should be on vegetables and fruits. A recent medical report on diet and the prevention of cancer looked at colorectal, prostate, stomach, esophagus, pancreas, and uterus cancers, and a summary of the recommendations are as follows:[52]

- Eat plenty of fruits and vegetables (at least five servings a day).
- Eat plenty of cereal foods, mainly in an unprocessed form.
- Maintain ideal body weight.
- Avoid fatty foods.
- Eat unprocessed red meat in moderation.
- Drink alcohol in moderation.
- Do not smoke.
- Avoid highly salted and moldy foods.
- Exercise regularly.
- Avoid eating chicken treated with antibiotics and hormones.

- Avoid eating burned or charred food.
- Avoid processed meats.
- Avoid processed fats such as margarine.
- Watch your sugar intake.

There has been some discussion that taking antioxidants together with chemotherapy decreases the effects of the chemotherapy cancer treatment. The consensus now, however, is that antioxidants improve the efficacy of both chemotherapeutic drugs and radiation,[53] and in addition, they also reduce the toxicity of anticancer drugs.[54] If you have cancer, however, it is important that you discuss any extra remedies with your medical doctor.

Environmental Chemicals and Pollutants

Some environmental chemicals are unavoidable. To offset these, I recommend that you do the following:

- Buy at least some organically grown foods. When I was a horticulture student, I visited various commercial farms and orchards and was shocked by the amount of chemicals used.
- Grow some green vegetables and herbs. Commercially grown green vegetables such as cabbage and lettuce are usually heavily sprayed with chemicals. Furthermore, certain beneficial antioxidants in plants degrade within twenty-four hours of harvesting.
- Exercise away from heavy traffic areas and get out of city pollution as often as possible.
- Keep household and garden chemicals to a minimum.

Supplements and Herbs

There are many theories and hopes but not many supportive scientific studies about the anticancer benefits of supplements and herbs, but, the following are worth mentioning:

- Omega-3 oil, 18 grams daily, plus 200 IU (135 milligrams) vitamin E, given to a group of terminal cancer patients extended survival rates, thought to be due to improved CD4/CD8 ratios (a measure of immune functioning).[55]
- Selenium supplementation benefited cancer patients on cisplatin-containing chemotherapy by reducing toxicity and improving kidney and immune function.[56]

Everyone can exercise, adjust their diet, improve their lifestyle, and take vitamin E and perhaps a multivitamin/mineral supplement. Take into consideration your other risk factors and get a practitioner's advice. At least for preventive purposes, these steps should form the core of your health strategies.

Chapter 10 concentrates on the emotional aspects of aging and menopause and developing an appropriate philosophy that doesn't involve pretending that you're going to live forever or ignoring the reality that your body will eventually wear out.

CHAPTER TEN

Menopause and Aging:
Strategies for Your Mind and Spirit

*P*ostmenopausal women's attitudes about "the change" are not nearly as negative as those who are approaching menopause, suggesting that the expectations are worse than the reality. Nevertheless, all change is relatively stressful, and because stress is inevitable in all our lives, we need strategies to avoid it, handle it, or overcome it.

Throughout this book, I emphasize the importance of diet and lifestyle but the way you think becomes more important as you age.

> We are what we think.
> All that we are arises with our thoughts.
> With our thoughts we make the world.
> Speak or act with a pure mind
> And happiness will follow you,
> Like an ever-present shadow.
>
> —*Buddha*

Despite a plethora of antiaging books and articles, aging is inevitable. Just as your bone cells get broken down so that they can be replaced with new ones, the human body wears out and other bodies come into existence. The same pattern happens in every living thing.

Perhaps the purpose of physical human aging is to make us aware of that part of our inner energy that does not age. If we stayed physically young we might focus only on the physical and possibly get bored with ourselves. Could an eighty-year-old mind cope with a twenty-year-old body? All that wisdom and all those hormones in combination might present serious conflicts!

Life is meant to be enjoyable. If you dwell on the physical, however, it is likely that your elderly life will be harder to enjoy because of reduced strength, lowered sex drive, joint weaknesses, and so on. Therefore, in very old age you may need to be more content with social, mental, and philosophical attainments.

When you gaze into a fire, see dolphins gliding through the water, look at a beautiful painting, sit quietly in a rainforest, or learn about the good deeds of others, something within you bubbles to the surface, and you experience some inexplicable emotion—that is your Spirit. Making the connection between the body, mind, and spirit requires conscious effort by you.

Buddha's last words were, "Find your own salvation." These words do not mean that you cannot seek help and guidance elsewhere, as long as you can discriminate between beneficial and inappropriate teachings.

There are many different paths and methods of connecting to the Spirit within you, such as:

- Antistress strategies
- Getting your brain to work for you, not against you
- Simplifying your life and your desires
- Mindfulness and concentration
- Prayer and religion
- Meditation

ANTISTRESS STRATEGIES

To feel or do anything, you need a body and mind, and they need to be looked after, along the lines of the previous chapters in this book.

Physical Exercise

Considerable evidence demonstrates that physical activities reduce anxiety, stress, and depression. Getting your body moving is necessary for good circulation, and your circulation carries oxygen and nutrients to every cell in the body, including the brain. Animal studies show that regular physical exercise increases nerve growth factor, which stimulates the production of new brain cells.

Yoga is an ideal activity that combines stretching, relaxation, breathing, and meditation. Stretching the muscles and then relaxing releases both physical and mental tension. Studies of disabled and disadvantaged people show that yoga can improve sleep, mental ability, social skills, and coordination as well as decrease substance abuse by strengthening willpower and reducing anxiety.[1]

Another study showed that when people were recovering from a heart attack they were better able to follow dietary and lifestyle changes if they did yogalike relaxation techniques, indicating that slowing down your mind actually increases willpower and allows you to come to grips with what is truly important.

Breathing

Slow, soothing, repetitive, and rhythmical activity will transmit relaxing stimuli to the brain; this in turn directs the muscles to relax. This activity should never be forced, so don't worry about restlessness or wandering thoughts. Breath is a key to relaxation. A simple technique follows: Let the breath flow in and out naturally and evenly. Visualize with each exhale that you are breathing out gray smoke, which represents your worries, aches and pains, and negative thoughts. After a few minutes, picture with each inhale that you are breathing in a gentle, healing energy. This energy could be in the form of a soft glowing light. Another option is simply to watch the breath flowing in and out, saying to yourself "breathing in, breathing out."

Some anxious people actually get worse if they focus on the breath, so they may need to use other techniques such as music or imagery.

Music

In a study of postoperative patients, music was more helpful than rest for pain and insomnia. One study found that classical music reduced tension; new age music decreased tension and hostility and increased relaxation (but also decreased vigor and mental clarity); and "designer music" increased caring, relaxation, mental clarity, and vigor and decreased hostility, fatigue, and tension. Grunge rock, on the other hand, increased hostility, sadness, tension, and fatigue and decreased caring, relaxation, vigor, and mental clarity.

Aromatherapy

Aromas have an effect on your nervous system. When women were asked to recall events brought to mind by neutral words such as "house" and "table" in conjunction with a discreet and pleasant fragrance, the result was happy memories. When the same words were used in conjunction with nasty smells, the result was unpleasant memories.

Aromatherapy is the art of using aromatic oils from plants to treat emotional and physical problems. Scientific studies have verified that odors are chemical messengers that have the capacity to modify our moods. When an odor rated as very pleasant is placed under the nostrils, increased bursts of electrical activity can be seen on the surface of the right hemisphere of the brain; shortly after the odor is removed, there is a similar burst of activity as if the brain were confirming that the experience had been pleasant.

Table 10.1 lists aromatic oils and their effects. The simplest way to use aromatic oils is to put a few drops on the back of the neck as a perfume.

Laughter Therapy

There's an old saying that, "A person without a sense of humor is like a wagon without springs—jolted by every stone on the road." Laughter has several benefits, including the following:

- Relieves stress
- Reduces blood pressure

TABLE 10.1 **Aromatic Oils and Their Effects**

Aromatic Oil	Effect
Bergamot	Antidepressant
Chamomile	Offsets lowness of spirit, restlessness, confusion, and insomnia
Clary sage	Enhances mental well-being and courage
Geranium	Balancing capacity during times of change and anxiety
Jasmine	Warming and stimulating
Lavender	Relaxing
Melissa	Mental tonic for the oversensitive
Rose	Antidepressant
Rosemary	Clarifies the mind

- Increases mucous excretion from the lungs
- Reduces pain
- Helps establish relationships
- Facilitates learning
- Relaxes muscles
- Tones the intestinal organs
- May help prevention and recovery from diseases
- Increases circulation

It has been demonstrated that after watching a movie that is a comedy, positive feelings and creative mental energy scores improve. For example, saliva samples were taken during a viewing of a humorous film and compared with samples taken during an academic film about anxiety. A biochemical compound known to prevent viruses was found to be higher during the viewing of the humorous film.[2]

How to Get More Laughter

- Only about 6 percent of laughter occurs when you are alone, so don't be too much of a homebody, especially if you live alone.

- Pets can be very amusing.
- Noncompetitive physical activity is frequently associated with laughter.
- Keep a joke file. When you hear a joke, make a point of remembering a few key words and the punch line.
- Instead of getting angry, try the following one-liners:

  "Let's not complicate our relationship by trying to communicate with each other."

  "The time for action is past—now is the time for senseless bickering."

  "I can't be bought—but make me an offer."

Colors

Studies in prisons and other institutions show that colors have an effect on behavior. You may find that colors you wear or look at can help you. See table 10.2.

TABLE 10.2 Colors and Their Effects on Behavior

Color	Effect
Red	Stimulating and warming. Good when you're feeling tired and dispirited. Not recommended for angry or confused people.
Orange	Brings tolerance and cheerfulness.
Yellow	Encourages optimism; helps increase mental alertness.
Green	Harmonizing and cleansing.
Blue	Calming and cooling.
Purple	For inspiration and intuition. Not good for people suffering from depression.
Violet	Tranquilizing; helps develop spirituality. Not recommended for those with low mental and physical energy.

Good Company

Find friends who have positive outlooks because stress is contagious. When unstressed rats are placed with stressed ones, the nontraumatized ones not only take on the stressed behavioral characteristics, but their blood chemistry changes as well. In my clinic I often see people who are suffering because of the stress of others; the consultation is with the wrong person! Once you are aware of the source of the stress, however, you may be able to use your own positive thoughts and actions to help offset this problem.

Is There a Medical Cause for Your Stress?

Stress can be linked to medical problems such as anemia, diabetes, or hormone imbalances. For example, if thyroid activity is too low, you will feel exhausted and unable to cope; if thyroid activity is too high, you will be in a state of agitation. If you don't eat properly, your blood sugar may be too low, which may cause shakiness. It's always wise to look for a medical cause because poor handling of stress can be linked to allergies, insomnia, and excessive alcohol intake.

Natural Antistress Remedies

Severe stress requires professional help. Day-to-day stress can be helped by remedies such as the following:

- Kava (not the alcoholic drink)
- Ginseng (the best antistress herb)
- B vitamin complex
- Vitamin C
- Skullcap, passion flower, and other relaxant herbs

Natural remedies and treatments for the brain are either tonics or relaxants, allowing you to sort out your problems better. There have been at least eighty scientific trials using herbs for depression, anxiety, and insomnia. In general, the results among many thousands of participants have been good to impressive, with side effects reported by less than 3 percent of patients.

Noninvasive antistress strategies include learning new skills, participating in social activities, intereacting with pets, maintaining spiritual practices, and helping other people. For instance, when people practiced transcendental meditation for four months, the effects of chronic stress were significantly reversed.[3]

GET YOUR BRAIN TO WORK FOR YOU, NOT AGAINST YOU

You have somewhere from 10 to 30 billion brain cells. Your brain cells need nutrients, oxygen, a nontoxic bloodstream, activity as well as rest, and various biochemicals. Every day, millions of messages are coded, sent, received, decoded, actioned, and stored.

Keeping your brain cells healthy requires the following:

- Good nutrition and circulation are essential because they carry fuel and oxygen for the brain.
- Physical and mental activity provide the stimuli to help keep the brain young.
- Your brain needs the time during sleep and relaxation to sort and file your thoughts.
- Train yourself to be a positive thinker. Believe that you can take an active role in your well-being.
- Natural therapy remedies and nondrug treatments can help your mental and emotional functioning.
- Avoid excessive alcohol and other harmful lifestyle choices that can damage your brain cells.

Maintaining optimal brain function also means that you should adhere to the following:

- Avoid putting yourself down, because this repetition gets recorded in your brain. Sometimes people say negative things about themselves and then get upset when others repeat it. There's already an overabundance of criticism in this world; don't add to it.

- Recognize your negative inner voice. Don't worry about it because none of us is perfect, but do make a conscious effort to be positive. Your thinking produces your feelings and leads to how you behave and react. There's an old Indian saying, "A man may have received the grace of God, of the teacher, and of holy men, but if he does not have the grace of his own mind he will go to rack and ruin."
- Stop dwelling in the past. You can't stop the birds of sadness from flying over you, but you can stop them from building nests in your hair.
- Ignore put-downs by other people. Sometimes put-downs are simply someone's habitual, unthinking way of making conversation and are not meant to be mean. Other people deflect their own problems by criticizing others. One way of handling put-downs is to avoid the person with the mean tongue; another is to visualize that the words are merely washing over you. Yet another strategy is to tell the person that the remarks are hurtful. Sometimes you can make people aware of their criticisms by complimenting them. As a last resort, you could take an assertiveness training course or teach yourself "tongue fu."

"Tongue fu" is the art of protecting yourself from verbal attacks. For example, if someone makes unfavorable comments about your appearance, you might try saying something like, "You should have seen me before the plastic surgery." If you're being ordered around unnecessarily, perhaps respond with "Does a bird in the sky need a path?" When you get tired of self-improvement advice, say, "I'm going to take the underachievers' course for very small business opportunities."

Don't blame yourself for traumas and diseases. Many of our circumstances are beyond our control, so don't make things worse by thinking that you deserved these calamities or they were caused by your personality traits.

The Power of Positive Thinking

Optimism is associated with a lower incidence of several diseases. A U.S. medical study over a thirty-year period showed that optimists experienced a 19 percent lower death rate compared with pessimists.[4] Various other studies have confirmed that pessimism increases the risk of a number of diseases and early death.

Optimists also recover better and are more active after coronary artery bypass surgery compared with those whose psychological profiles indicated low optimism. I've observed in my own clinic that people who cope well with severe illnesses often say things like, "I'm quite healthy except for the cancer and diabetes." Others feel that a minor upset is ruining their lives.

SIMPLIFY YOUR LIFE

Aside from wanting peace and happiness, modern life seems to encourage high expectations and a great desire for possessions and pleasures. Yet when we achieve the things we desire, are we content, or are we afraid of losing them? Do we want even more? Are other people then envious or even enraged? As Buddha said, "Even if it rained gold, you would not be satisfied." Although self-improvement is part of human nature, we all need to develop a philosophy that allows us to be relatively content.

When the mind dwells on the pleasures of the senses,
Attraction arises for those pleasures.
From attraction arises desire to obtain them.
When you can't get them, anger arises.
Anger leads to confusion in the mind.
When your mind is confused you lose your memory and reasoning
    powers.
When you lose your memory and reasoning, you are lost.
                              —Adapted from Bhagavad Gita

MINDFULNESS

Most Eastern philosophies and religions emphasize mindfulness and focusing on the present. We all learn from the past, and it is good to be hopeful and have goals. If you dwell on the past, however, you are going over lost time; and if you dwell on the future, you are postponing happiness or living in vain hope. How can you be sure that another place or another time will be better?[5]

In my clinic I sometimes see people in their seventies who still feel bitter about some real or imagined sin that was inflicted on them decades ago. There is some evidence that bad memories can lead to illness. In a series of carefully controlled experiments, rats were given a toxic chemical substance flavored with saccharine. Later, when they were given only saccharine-flavored water, they had the same gastric discomfort and suppressed immune function as experienced from the toxins. In other words, their association with the unpleasant past experience actually made them physically ill.

How to Be Mindful

To begin, you can practice mindfulness for part of each day or part of each week. Don't do tasks just to get them over with. Do each activity in a relaxed way with your full attention. Do the task in a measured fashion, without reluctance. Mindfulness does not have any element of judging, just observing. You might observe your thoughts, for example. Just as you are not to judge yourself, avoid judging others; judging is a bad habit that leads to resentment and anxiety.

Whenever your mind becomes scattered, say to yourself "Breathing in, breathing out." One system of meditation is simply to observe the breath; another is to focus on the middle of the forehead and imagine that you are taking in energy from that point.

The breath can be used to focus the mind and develop wisdom. Once you know how to use the breath, it can help you overcome difficulties. Your breath is the bridge from your body to your mind and makes possible oneness of body and mind. When you are at peace, your breath is part of the energy source. When you have achieved mindfulness, you will be peaceful and look at others with an open mind and fondness.

In one scientifically controlled study, a mindfulness meditation technique was used, and the researcher concluded that psychological symptoms improved and that participants had achieved a greater sense of control or acceptance as well as spiritual experiences.[6]

.ar as I know, no one is certain where your thoughts actually come
. Be aware of your thoughts without worrying about them, however,
.ause the mind is like a monkey, swinging from branch to branch. To not
lose sight of the monkey, we must watch it constantly.

PRAYER AND RELIGION

Some Christian Experiences

In a controlled trial of 496 patients, prayer resulted in significant improvements in self-esteem, anxiety, and depression.[7] Similarly, a scientific survey
showed that those who attended a religious service once a week, prayed daily,
or studied the Bible daily were 40 percent less likely to have high blood pressure than those who did so less often.[8] Socializing with like-minded people
or some form of regular contact appeared to be an important factor.

Although contemplation has always been important in monasteries,
daily meditation is now rediscovered as part of the Christian tradition.
Gerald Searle recommends that you be "on the journey" and that you commit yourself to the daily discipline. It is a lifelong commitment. It is about
union with God as you know God. It calls for discipline, patience, commitment, perseverance, and generosity.

One of the suggestions in Searle's book, *Stillness Be My Friend*, is the following mantra: *Maranatha*, an Aramaic word meaning, "Come, Lord." Say it
in four equally stressed syllables: ma-ra-na-tha. Say it from the beginning to
the end of the meditation. Sound it, listen to it. With time, the mantra will
sound itself, it will become your friend, your source of immeasurable peace
and wisdom. It will become your closest and lifelong companion.[9]

A Scientist's View

The late Roger J. Williams, a distinguished biochemist, researcher, and
author of *You Are Extraordinary*, wrote that it is wholly beyond human intellectual powers to truly understand God, but that does not mean that God
does not exist. Just as there are many facets to human minds, there are prob-

ably many facets to God. Williams cited music, creativity, and the concern that we have for other people as a few of those aspects of God.

In Williams's Utopia Game, players were given a list of fifty things, including marriage, gardening, athletics, eating, conversation, odors, reading, and religious worship. They were told to imagine that they were on a journey to their ideal place and that each of these fifty things was to be considered as a piece of baggage. On the boat trip, however, they encountered heavy seas, and some of the baggage had to be dumped. Everyone had to rank the things in order of importance. There was a wide variety in preferences, but the striking feature was that religious worship rated the highest overall.

In assessing how individuals value religion, Dr. Williams concluded that: "When the inborn individuality of people is fully recognized, there will be no more search for the one true interpretation of God and there will be no cause for distrusting those who do not believe just as we do. When students are taught to appreciate the individuality of their minds, they will be able to choose in the field of religion, without friction, whatever suits them best. Very few, under these conditions, will choose irreligion."[10]

The Wisdom of the Dalai Lama[11]

Altruism: Acting for the Good of Others You want to be happy and other people want to be happy, and we are all dependent on the cooperation, help, and kindness of others. No one makes friends through confrontation, insults, or hatred. In the next life, a favorable birth is attained if we restrain from actions that are harmful to others.

Recognizing the Enemy Your own jealousy, attachment, fear, anger, and hatred are your real enemies. Negative states of mind obscure intelligence and judgment. When you are faced with adverse circumstances, feeling unhappy serves no purpose in overcoming the problem. If someone was the cause of the problem, your sad attitude may cause that person delight or encouragement.

Overcoming the Enemy The main causes of anger are dissatisfaction, fear, and unhappiness, and these feelings disturb your peace of mind.

People want happiness, but they engage in activities that lead to suffering. If someone harms you, will your anger change his essential nature? If someone is preventing you from getting something you want, ask whether you will truly benefit from that particular thing. If you feel envious, your envy will not affect others; instead of being unhappy you should be glad of the success of others. To develop, you need someone to test you. The more selfish and self-centered you are, the more lonely and miserable you become. Observe for yourself. With practice, the mind can be trained. Think that you will help others in proper ways. If that is not possible, at least do not harm others.

MEDITATION

Even one who wishes to learn meditation rises above those who merely follow instructions.

—Bhagavad Gita

The word *meditation* was first coined as *dhyana* (in Sanskrit) thousands of years ago and was part of the ancient yogic system of becoming one with the Creator.

Stress management or relaxation therapy may be considered a form of meditation. In the traditional sense, however, meditation was designed to help find the spirit within yourself so that a person could become aware of the Creator in everything. Consequently, the meditator could achieve fearlessness, calm, and contentment. There's an old yogic saying that "the first sign of spirituality is cheerfulness," so if you are joining a meditation group and the teacher and students look miserable, you might try another system!

If you want to meditate, you first have to learn how to relax. In this context relaxation can be considered a state of serene alertness: anything that makes you feel calm is relaxation. Once you are reasonably calm, you can begin to concentrate on one thing and then you can meditate. The benefits of meditation include the following:

- Prevents premature aging
- Has antioxidant effects on lipids

- Reduces the effects of stress
- Increases brain blood flow
- Lowers blood pressure and cholesterol
- Improves memory and learning ability
- Assists abstract reasoning and intelligence
- Heightens creativity and sense perception
- Reduces asthma symptoms
- Helps immune functioning
- Improves cardiovascular efficiency
- Improves self-esteem
- Beneficial effects in personal relationships
- Reduces depression
- May help reduce addictions
- Leads to spiritual awareness

A study of long-term transcendental meditation practitioners showed that they had 15 percent less lipid peroxides in their blood compared with a control group.[12] Lipid peroxides are potentially harmful oxidized fats that are linked to atherosclerosis, heart disease, cancer, and premature aging. An evaluation of 423 experienced practitioners of transcendental meditation found they had significantly higher levels of DHEA than non-meditators.[13] DHEA is an adrenal hormone that many researchers consider to be a marker of aging, although some exaggerated claims are suggesting that DHEA in the form of a pill is an elixir of youth. A DHEA pill can have adverse effects, whereas the amount generated by meditation and exercise is beneficial.

Meditation improves hearing, vision, learning, and reaction time and reduces blood pressure. In addition, surveys indicate that meditators have reduced medical utilization rates for sixteen of seventeen major medical treatment categories, including 55.4 percent fewer hospital admissions for tumors and 87 percent fewer admissions for heart disease compared with those who did not meditate.[14] These findings could also mean that people who take up meditation are more health conscious than nonmeditators.

Meditation Techniques

Taking a course is probably the best way to learn about meditation because you can ask questions and adapt many of the teachings to suit your own beliefs and temperament. You may have to try a few different systems before you find what suits you. In my yoga classes I teach mainly yogic meditation, but the majority of my Roman Catholic students simply adapt the teaching to their own beliefs. Some common meditation techniques include the following:

- Symbols and visualization
- Sounds
- Thoughts and themes
- Developing an unforced rhythmic breathing pattern
- Guided imagery

For beginners, I suggest starting with about ten minutes of meditation a day and gradually working up to twenty or thirty minutes once or twice daily. Forcing yourself into long periods of meditation when you are involved in everyday modern life is like trying to put a car in reverse when you are traveling at high speed.

Some people end up worrying about not being able to sit still, let alone meditate. It is quite difficult, so even if you start sitting calmly for ten minutes and have a few minutes of concentration within that time, that is a starting point. You might discover that if you tell yourself to be still and not to think, the urge to fidget and think will be even greater. Conversely, if you aim to concentrate on your thoughts, your mind may become blank!

Sit in any comfortable position but aim for good posture; be upright, relaxed, and alert. Think of the meditation exercise as a holiday from your everyday pressures. Some people do minimeditations throughout the day to offset stress or to remind themselves of their spiritual indweller. For example, calmly observe the breath for a few minutes or repeat a mantra.

It doesn't matter if you're not very good at the meditation exercises; even very experienced meditators go through times when they cannot concentrate.

Following are a few examples of techniques suitable for beginners.

Symbols and Visualization as Meditation Techniques Visualize a light with the eyes closed.

Picture a tiny soft white glowing light within the heart, or outside the body between the eyebrow center. At the same time, you could silently and slowly repeat a verse, such as

I meditate on the light of the Creator
That permeates and sustains the universe
And glows within all living beings
May this light enlighten me
And direct me to the Truth.
　—Adaptation of the Gayatri Mantra

Sounds (Mantras) A mantra is a sound, word, phrase, or verse with spiritual significance. In Sanskrit the word itself means "that which protects." There are many hundreds of mantras in the yogic tradition; they were discovered by spiritually advanced monks during periods of deep meditation. Mantras can be repeated silently or out loud.

An easy technique for beginners is to sit calmly and repeat silently the word *shanti* (pronounced shon-tee), meaning "peace." Specific mantras are given by spiritual teachers to students, but there are some universal mantras such as the Gayatri mantra above that are usually recited in Sanskrit.

Thoughts The lotus flower is a common symbol in Eastern philosophies and religions. You could calmly gaze at a picture of a lotus flower or water lily, thinking about the symbolism of it growing in the mud but not being sullied by the dirt, or repeat the following verse:

In the heart center of our bodies
There is a small shrine in the form of a lotus flower

And within there is a tiny space
We should find out what is in that tiny space
And we should try to understand it
And if anyone should ask
What is in that tiny space within the lotus of the heart?
We can answer
In that tiny space is a whole universe
For IT is everywhere and IT is within us
And if anyone should ask
What happens when old age overtakes us
And the body is no more?
We can answer
The tiny space within the lotus of the heart
Is not touched by fire or water
IT is beyond sorrow, old age and death
IT is Atman, it is pure spirit.

—Adapted from Chandogya Upanishad

Meditation on Breath

Regular breathing puts the body in a harmonious condition and
then it is easier to reach the mind.

—Swami Vivekananda

A number of meditation systems place emphasis on breathing. There are
some complicated breathing techniques, but to begin with I advise people
to find their own natural breathing rhythm, inhaling and exhaling at the
same pace. In yoga, breathing techniques are called *pranayama*, but *prana* is not
simply breathing, but represents the source of all energy.

Try the following:

1. As you breathe in, say to yourself the word *om*.
2. As you breathe out, count from I to 108.

These steps are done to your natural breathing rhythm. If you lose count, just become aware of your lack of concentration, guess what number you had reached, and continue. Once you are comfortable and able to reach 108, do two rounds.

Guided Meditation I suggest recording the following on audio tape. Say it slowly and allow time for each phrase to be repeated silently, while imagining the scene.

I picture a large range of mountains, like the Himalayas. Below the high peaks, the snow is slowly melting and forming tiny, gushing streams. Further down the mountains, the little streams begin to merge, forming a stream that cascades and tumbles downward, cutting its way through the hills. The water is uncontrolled and swiftly flowing. Nothing can tame it.

Eventually, the water reaches the plains and becomes a slow-flowing river, meandering toward the ocean. This river represents my controlled self. The river reaches the coast, slows down and widens, eventually dissolving into the ocean.

Where does the water originate? Some say in the mountains, but it actually originates in the ocean. The life-giving sun causes the water to evaporate. The evaporated water gets into the clouds, and the clouds form the snow and rain that fall on the mountains and hills.

The water rushing down from the mountains and hills is like my mind. When I am engaged in everyday activities, the mind is often uncontrolled, with thoughts rushing in from everywhere. At least for a few minutes each day, I will think of myself as the ocean. I am not like a boat being pounded by the waves and wind. I am engaged in activity but not affected by everything that is going on around me.

The ancient sages tell us that just as all waters originate in the ocean, fall from the sky, and ultimately return to the ocean, so all beings originate from and return to the Creator. When I am my calm, wise self, I think of myself as the ocean. On the surface there are waves and all sorts of activities, but nothing disturbs the depths of the ocean. It is vast and calm. I become part of that vast stillness. I can take part in everyday life like the activity on the surface of the ocean, but deep down I am calm and peaceful.

Is Meditation Helpful for Everyone? A few people who suffer from severe anxiety, panic attacks, and depression may become worse if they force themselves to sit in silence. They need professional counseling and then some relaxation and concentration techniques before trying meditation.

Antistress strategies and positive thinking can improve your physical and emotional well-being. Mindfulness enables you to live fully, and meditation is a way of handling stress, avoiding premature aging, and dealing with old age. Strive to become wiser with age so that the mind and the spirit become more important than the body.

CHAPTER ELEVEN

Sex: A Necessity or an Optional Extra?

wo elderly ladies were at a senior citizens' get-together. At the end of the meeting, the hostess passed around a tray of cheese and wine, which prompted the local minister to say in a loud voice, "I would rather commit adultery than drink alcohol." One of the ladies put her glass of wine back on the tray and said to her friend, "I didn't know we had a choice."

You may have already discovered that having a satisfying and active sex life is not simply a matter of choice. For about 50 percent of post-menopausal women, giving advice to have an active sex life is simply unrealistic, for a number of reasons.

Women live longer than men. In the United States, the average man lives to age seventy-three, whereas the average female lives to seventy-nine. In most developed countries, there are about twice as many women as men at age eighty-five and over. And, the vast majority of older women are heterosexual.

Furthermore, most sex occurs in the home, so if you're living alone, you're at a disadvantage. In most developed countries, there are almost three times as many women over sixty living alone compared with men. Over age seventy-five, only about one-fifth of women are living with a partner.

Sexual functioning is more difficult for aging men than women, which means that the scarce resource (older men) has a lowered capacity. Although various injections and drugs are now available, they have potential side effects. First, older men can put their hearts under stress if they have too much sexual activity, particularly if they are physically unfit. Second, if a pill is taken to maintain an erection for a long period of time, the woman's vagina tissue may not be strong enough, assuming the older man has a partner in his own age group.

Although some women like to think of themselves as forever young and desirable, others fit more comfortably into a grandmotherly role. A typical married couple in their early fifties have probably had sexual intercourse about 3,000 times, so they might not be as enthusiastic as they were thirty years earlier.

MIDDLE AGE AND SEXUALITY

Although there is a gradual decrease in sexual interest and activity with age for both men and women, many are sexually active into midlife and beyond. This decrease is not always the same between partners, however, which can be a problem. Danish women aged fifty-one reported no change in sexual desire, and, surprisingly, the researchers said that there was a significant correlation between hormone replacement therapy and decreasing desire.[1] Most of the women I see in my clinic who are on HRT tell me that the hormones improve their sex life, but that may be due to a reduction of hot flashes and sweating, which in turn improves well-being.

In another survey of postmenopausal women, 51 percent reported that their partners had decreased sexual interest; it was also revealed that 49 percent had difficulty achieving an erection, 44 percent had difficulty maintaining an erection, 24 percent had premature ejaculation, and 17 percent had delayed ejaculation. It is not surprising that 56 percent of the women had difficulty with lubrication, 56 percent reported diminished sexual arousal, 44 percent reported a lack of orgasm, and 25 percent reported decreased vaginal sensation.[2] Interestingly, women report high levels of partners' lack of interest, whereas the men do not report it. Obviously, men who are having erectile and ejaculatory problems may shun intercourse even though desire does not wane.

Aside from natural and normal hormonal changes, many other things are happening at midlife. It's not easy for most women to switch "on" to sex, especially if they're worried about their husband's health, parents' lack of independence, or their "baby" is getting married. In addition, you may be evaluating your changing role in the workplace and home. These types of stresses can dampen sexual interest and behavior.

Menopausal and postmenopausal women who are in stable relationships commonly say that they would prefer to be sexually active. They do, though, find it difficult to talk about their needs in an explicit way with their partners because it has never been a subject for unabashed, honest discussion. Given that older women need more arousal time to get vaginal lubrication, they need to discuss this need. Some difficulties may be overcome by changing a couple's typical sexual repertoire or by counseling.

Is Hormone Therapy Necessary for an Active Sex Life?

Sexual functioning is widely variable. Physical symptoms, general health, psychological well-being, economic and social status, family issues, partner's physical and psychological state, and communication all affect quality of life and greatly affect sexuality. Sexual desire usually plummets when women are not emotionally attached to their partners or if they are upset about something. Body image, general health, and even beliefs about menopause and sexuality affect sexual functioning.[3] Researchers found that there were no differences between HRT users and nonusers regarding negative mood and sexual desire.[4]

In a poll of 100 healthy, married, menopausal women (before HRT became commonly prescribed), 65 percent maintained that there was no change in their sexuality. Of the remainder, half thought sexual activity became less important and half thought sexual relations became more enjoyable.[5]

My interpretation of the evidence is that lack of sexual activity is commonly associated with scarcity of men, ego, marital problems, social circumstances, stress, and ill health. Aging and hormones are only two of the factors.

Dutch researchers reported that complaints of vaginal dryness and difficult intercourse seem to reflect a sexual arousal problem rather than vaginal shrinking associated with menopause. They reported that "no significant relationship was found between hormones and sexual function."[6] Most reports from various countries advise that there is a decline in sexual response and activity in postmenopausal women, but that decline is related to many factors. The research cited in this chapter highlights the mistake of linking every problem to menopause. Postmenopausal women, however, need a longer arousal time, which may be difficult when their partners are also having their own problems with achieving or sustaining an erection.

Hormone replacement therapy doesn't make bad relationships good, nor will it miraculously improve your social and self-worth status. In some cases it may be that in middle age a woman simply refuses to continue with bad or selfish sex.

IS SEX ESSENTIAL?

In a sense, sex is essential; otherwise, there would be no living beings. Yet various surveys show that almost one-third of healthy women, from teenagers to the elderly, are not sexually active, and, as you would expect, most of them are single or elderly.[7] Common sexual problems reported included inhibition or anxiety and lack of sexual pleasure. In older women a lack of lubrication and painful intercourse was reported, although it was not a major problem.

Sex is not entirely essential for day-to-day functioning, and many people get along without it. If you're accustomed to it, however, it's not easy to go without it. Men, unfortunately, die sooner than women and have a high level of sexual problems as they age. Others may leave their middle-aged wives, sometimes for younger women. I don't have much to offer except to say that you won't find a replacement, or good company, if you mope around the house. The only way to preserve your dignity is to participate in different social activities that interest you. You will then, I hope, meet compatible people of both sexes.

If you haven't the opportunity or the desire for an active sex life, you're in good company. There are drives nobler than sex, and many people lead celibate and rewarding lives without retiring into a religious order. Germaine Greer summed it up very well by concluding that: "Despite all the evidence to show that celibates are no madder and often a good deal healthier than the rest of the population, they (menopause doctors) persist in the irrational belief that regular psychosexual release is essential for the proper functioning of all individuals."[8]

In my practice, I see a number of elderly couples who have not had sex for years, and they seem adjusted and content. Although some older couples may have a good sex life, for others mature love doesn't necessarily hinge on the ability to make the bedsprings creak.

LIBIDO AND ANDROGENS

There is an increasing trend to prescribe testosterone (a male hormone) to women with low libido, but because this hormone produces male characteristics, many women are reluctant to use it. As table 11.1 shows, it seems that testosterone not estrogen is higher in sexually active older women.

There does not seem to be any connection between female hormones and increased female sexual activity. A British study found that an enzyme that

TABLE 11.1 Hormone Levels of Women Aged Sixty to Seventy		
	Sexually active	*Sexually inactive*
Number of women	31.0	18.0
Female hormones:		
Estradiol (ng/mL)	7.6	9.4
Luteinizing hormone (miu/mL)	59.0	68.0
Male hormones:		
Bound testosterone (ng/dL)	268.0	203.0
Free testosterone (ng/dL)	1.42	1.19

Source: G. S. Bachmann and S. R. Leiblum, "Sexuality in Sexagenerian Women," *Maturitas* 13 (1991): 46.

Note: A nanogram (ng) is a measurement in billionths.

converts testosterone to a more active form is linked to sexual interest in post-menopausal women.[9] Although testosterone replacement (menopausal androgen replacement therapy) *may* increase libido and is being increasingly prescribed, a U.S. study of 130 women with breast cancer found results consistent with the theory that testosterone has an indirect effect on breast cancer via its influence on the amount of estrogen in the body.[10]

One researcher suggested that with aging we produce fewer pheromones (hormone-like chemicals that are like an invisible cloud around us). We are not conscious of these pheromones, but they are thought to enhance libido and contribute to a person's natural scent and attractiveness to the opposite sex.[11] This researcher considers that estrogen helps the brain and lymph and stimulates pheromones, thus contributing to the perception of female sex identity.

VAGINAL PROBLEMS

Like everything else, a menopausal vagina is not the same as a twenty-year-old one. The skin loses its tone, and the area loses a degree of elasticity. A baby's head would present extreme difficulty, although not the average penis.

A dry, itchy vagina is a problem for some menopausal and post-menopausal women, and it can make sex difficult and painful. A Swedish survey, however, showed that the most common reasons for not having a regular sex life were lack of a partner and lack of desire.[12] Only 4 percent stated that local vaginal discomfort was the main reason.

Causes of Vaginal Dryness

Vaginal dryness is caused by low levels of estrogen, and internal and external estrogens often alleviate the problem. One study has shown that women with the least vaginal degeneration had significantly higher levels of male hormones.[13] Male hormones make the skin "tougher" and generally stimulate sexual desire and arousal. The problem is that if these hormones are relatively high, they may also increase the growth of facial hair and produce other masculine characteristics, including aggressiveness.

Treatment

Estriol is weaker and probably safer than other estrogens. Studies indicate that it is helpful for vaginal dryness and may prevent recurring urinary tract infections in postmenopausal women.[14] Continued sexual activity has been found to protect against vaginal dryness.[15]

Vegetarian menopausal women seem to have fewer vaginal problems than nonvegetarians, irrespective of their sex life. A few scientific studies have confirmed that vaginal tissue was improved after only a few weeks of eating relatively small quantities of phytoestrogenic foods.

Some herbs, taken orally, may be helpful to increase vaginal lubrication and to reduce anxiety. These herbs are:

- Asian ginseng (Panax ginseng and Panax notoginseng)
- Dong quai
- Galangal (*Alpinia galanga*), a spicy herb that is similar to ginger. It can be purchased in Asian stores in powder form and used on food. Take 1 to 2 teaspoons daily.

Depending on your symptoms, it may help to follow the menus outlined in chapter 3.

Some natural remedies, such as vitamin E oil, can be applied externally; these remedies are explained in chapter 5. I do not recommend petroleum-based products because although they may provide instant lubrication, if used frequently they seem to irritate vaginal skin.

If natural remedies do not give quick relief, I recommend practitioner advice and perhaps a prescription for estriol cream. This cream seems to be effective and probably has the least adverse reactions of all the hormonal medications.

Declining sexual activity is natural with aging, and sex problems may be related to dysfunction on the part of either partner.

Remember that various psychological, physical, social, and hormonal factors affect your sexual function. At the same time, HRT will not offset relationship and social problems.

If you are among the 50 percent of older women without a partner—or opportunities for regular sex—get out of the mental bind that you are not complete or completely alive unless you are sexually active. There are many other joyful and rewarding human experiences.

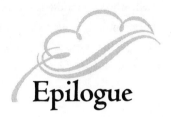

Epilogue

*M*enopause is not a disease, but a transition. Although our bodies become less efficient with age, it is possible to become physically and emotionally healthier by following these guidelines:

- As much as possible, identify the cause of emotional and physical problems and then do something now to overcome, contend with, or offset them.
- Eat correctly. It has been shown repeatedly that a diet rich in fruits and vegetables as well as whole grains, legumes, and fish provides antioxidants and compounds that help prevent premature aging and diseases.
- Get plenty of physical and mental exercise.
- Without being fanatical, avoid harmful foods and lifestyle habits.
- Avoid drugs as much as possible.
- Appropriate natural remedies can reduce the effects of many common ailments. If you treat them early, they are less likely to develop into something more severe.

- Train yourself to be a positive thinker.
- Learn to relax or practice meditation.
- Participate in religious or spiritual activities.

With all this information and advice, you may still not know how to proceed. You could start with some of the simple recommendations such as adding one new food or recipe a week. Or, you might begin with the problem that is causing you the most distress. Alternatively, seek help from a qualified health practitioner.

200 Reasons Not to Take
Hormone Replacement Therapy

*S*ome of the cautions and adverse reactions listed here may be somewhat theoretical and more likely to occur with stronger contraceptive hormone pharmaceuticals, but they are listed in a major pharmaceutical reference text indicating that there is at least a potential problem in sensitive people.

Possibly all the effects associated with oral contraceptives may occur with HRT, although they would be more subtle and over a longer term, at which time it may be difficult to distinguish these from the effects of aging.

Many of the problems associated with HRT in Australian texts are not listed in the United States; conversely, a few are listed in the United States but not in Australia. The difference is likely due to publishers, physicians, pharmaceutical companies, and government regulations, perhaps indicating an overall lack of agreement.

Prescriptions are for one to three different hormones and not the whole range, so any one individual would not be exposed to all the listed problems. A significant number of women, however, have been on almost lifelong oral contraceptives and may have used various types over the years. Menopausal women, too, may have taken a number of different regimes.

It is useful to have this list so that you can check symptoms for yourselves, which is why I have listed all the problems under all the categories.

Where the same problem has been listed as a contraindication, warning, and adverse reaction and where the problems occur under both estrogens and progestins, I have listed the problem under the various headings but counted it once only. A general warning, such as for cardiovascular disorders, has been counted once, but specific conditions such as hypertension have been counted separately.

To avoid double counting, those items listed for the second or third time have been marked with an asterisk and are not counted in the total. A few side issues have also been marked with an asterisk and not counted.

The two main reference texts used to compile the following lists are: A. Caswell (managing ed.), *MIMS Annual*, 23d edition, St. Leonards, NSW, MediMedia Australia Pty. Ltd., 1999 and USPDI, *Drug Information for the Health Care Professional*, 18th edition, vol. I, Rockville, Maryland, United States Pharmacopeial Convention Inc., 1998.

LIST 1
Estrogen pharmaceuticals: contraindications
REASONS I THROUGH 23:

- Cancer of the breast
- Nonhysterectomized women unless on progestin
- Undiagnosed vaginal bleeding
- Severe liver damage
- Current or past clotting disorders
- Current or past thrombosis
- Cerebrovascular (brain/circulation) disorders
- Cardiovascular (heart/circulation) disorders
- Lipid (fat) metabolism disturbances
- Known pregnancy
- Suspected pregnancy

- Otosclerosis (inner ear thickening), if deterioration occurred during pregnancy
- History of pruritis (itching)
- Herpes during pregnancy or from previous use of steroids
- Breast pathology
- Endometriosis
- Acute liver disease
- Chronic liver disease
- Past history of cholestatic jaundice
- Stroke history
- Sickle-cell anemia
- Severe uncontrolled hypertension
- High lipoproteins

LIST 2

Estrogen pharmaceuticals: warnings and precautions

REASONS 24 THROUGH 64:

- To be prescribed only after a thorough general medical and gynecological examination, including pap smear,* breast check,* blood pressure,* abdomen,* pelvic organs* and family history.*
- Periodic medical examination necessary every six to twelve months. Watch for:
  Unusual upper abdominal complaints
  Tetany (muscle spasm)
  Otosclerosis* (inner ear problem)
  Breakthrough bleeding
  Hypertension*
  Multiple sclerosis
  Endometrial cancer
  Uterine Cancer
  Breast pain
- Strict medical supervision and regular monitoring for worsening or triggering of:

Fibroids
Endocrine, cardiac,* kidney, or liver* dysfunction
Gallstones
Asthma
History of phlebitis (inflamed veins)
Epilepsy
Porphyria (inherited blood disorder)
Hepatic adenoma (liver tumor)
Gallbladder disease
Diabetes
Varicose veins
Embolism (clot or air bubble)
Chorea (twitching)
Depression

- Discontinue at earliest signs of thrombolic disorders (blood clots),* cerebrovascular disorders,* pulmonary embolism.*
- Due to danger of thrombosis, discontinue four to eight weeks prior to surgery.
- Cigarette smoking increases the risk of serious cardiovascular effects from the use of estrogens.
- Use care in patients with diseases affecting calcium and phosphorous metabolism.
- These pharmaceuticals may cause high blood calcium levels and may increase cortisol and thyroxine binding globulin (a thyroid protein).
- Discontinue if there is sudden, partial, or complete loss of vision or if there is sudden onset of proptosis (abnormal bulging or drooping of the eye) or double vision.
- Discontinue if there is migraine or hearing disturbances.
- Implants must be removed if liver function* is abnormal or if there is breast pain and increased cervical mucus.
- Estrogen drugs can affect the action of other drugs, and some drugs can affect estrogens and progestins. (Refer any questions to your health practitioner.) The effect of patches has not yet been fully evaluated in this respect.

- The possible benefits of long-term treatment need to be weighed against the risks.
- Dose should never exceed recommendations.* (This advice applies to everything.)

LIST 3

Estrogen pharmaceuticals: adverse reactions

REASONS 65 THROUGH 105:

- External side effects:
  Skin rashes
  Allergic reactions
  Spots or lumps
  Irritation, especially from patches
  Dark or red pigmentation
  Sensitivity to light
  Acne
  Loss of scalp hair
- Internal side effects:
  Nausea
  Bloating
  Vomiting
  Gallstones*
  Breakthrough bleeding*
  Period pain
  Vaginitis
  Increase in size of fibroids*
  Change in vaginal secretions*
  PMS-like symptoms
  Changes in libido
  Unwanted hair growth
  Migraine*
  Depression*
  Dizziness

Irritability
Mood changes
Weight change
Reduction in glucose tolerance*
Rise in blood pressure*
Palpitations
Musculoskeletal and bone pain
Fluid retention
Intolerance to contact lenses
Abdominal pain/cramps*
Anorexia
Jaundice
Changes in liver enzymes*
Change in menstrual flow
Pain on urination
Undersirable uterine growth
Reactivation of endometriosis*
Cystitis-like syndrome
Low doses may stimulate breast tumors*
Breast swelling/tenderness/secretions
Porphyria cutanea (liver/skin pigmentation)
Headaches
Nervousness
Fatigue
Neuritis (nerve pain)
Increased appetite
Rise in blood sugar*
Sodium and nitrogen retention
Thrombosis and other clotting disorders*
Worsening of varicose veins*
Spasms
Steepening of corneal curve

Note: Some women are prescribed HRT even though they are still menstruating.

The following apparent peculiarities are all taken from *MIMS Annual,* the main Australian pharmaceutical reference text. This text provides much more detail than the equivalent U.S. references. Premarin, Ogen, Estigyn, and Duphaston are the brand names of the drugs.

LIST 4

Specific anomalies: estrogen and progestin pharmaceuticals

REASONS 106 THROUGH 117:

These reasons seem to contradict current prescribing practices and publicity.

- There is no evidence of the minimum duration of estrogen replacement therapy for younger postmenopausal women which will be effective subsequently in reducing fracture at the age of greatest fracture risk at seventy-five years of age—Estraderm (estradiol patch)
- There is no evidence that estrogens are effective for nervous symptoms or depression without associated vasomotor symptoms and they should not be used to treat such conditions—Premarin
- For menopause symptoms, the lowest dose should be used for the shortest time—Premarin
- Large doses of estrogen (conjugated estrogens 5 mg/day) have been shown in a large prospective clinical trial (in men) to increase the risk of nonfatal heart attack—Premarin
  Note: Some women I see are on an even higher dose.
- Vitamin A plasma increases, B_{12} and vitamin C decrease—Ogen (estropipate)
- Leukocytes and thrombocytes decrease but the clinical significance is not known—Ogen
- Plasma triglycerides, phospholipids, LDL and VLDL may be increased—Ogen
  Note: Excess levels of these fats are harmful.
- May be an increased incidence of heart attacks in women over forty—Ogen

- While knowledge of the pharmokinetics of synthetic sex steroids is increasing, current knowledge is still fragmentary—Ogen
- Leaflet to be distributed to patient—Estigyn (ethinylestradiol) *Note:* In Australia, very few women are given either a comprehensive leaflet or full information. In the United States there is a mandatory patient package insert.
- Any possible influence of prolonged dydrogesterone therapy on pituitary, ovarian, hepatic, or uterine function awaits further study—Duphaston

LIST 5

Anomalies: problems listed in U.S. pharmaceutical reference text but not in Australia

REASONS 118 THROUGH 129:

- Pancreatitis may worsen or reoccur.
- Estrogens do not replace previously lost bone or significantly increase total bone mass.
- Elimination of estrogens is more prolonged in obese patients than in nonobese patients.
- Take with or immediately after food to reduce nausea. (The Australian recommendation is to take at the same time each day.)
- There is a possibility of dental problems, such as tenderness, swelling, or bleeding of the gums.
- The list of altered laboratory and biopsy values is much longer in the United States. Hence, if you have a blood test or tissue biopsy, the readings may be increased or decreased due to the HRT.
- Counseling women without symptoms about the risks and benefits is complex. The true estimates for long-term risks and benefits await controlled clinical trials.
- The U.S. pharmacopeial information is that the overall effect on bone density for progestins has yet to be established and may depend on type of progestin, dose, sex, and age of patient.

Vaginal Estrogens   Generally, vaginal estrogens are absorbed into the body at about 25 to 40 percent less than an estradiol tablet, so the basic warnings and potential adverse effects are similar to tablets. Some specific cautions in respect of vaginal estrogens are the following:

- Avoid exposing a male partner to estrogen vaginal cream.
- Do not use latex condoms for up to seventy-two hours after vaginal treatment because oils in the vaginal cream may weaken latex products.
- This product may cause vaginal discomfort, pain, or ulceration.

LIST 6
Progestin pharmaceuticals: contraindications
REASONS 130 THROUGH 133:

- Past or present thrombotic disorder*
- Past or present coronary artery disease*
- Undiagnosed breast pathology*
- Known or suspected pregnancy*
  Note: Causes birth anomalies.
- History of herpes during pregnancy*
- History of severe itching during pregnancy*
- Markedly impaired liver function*
- Dubin-Johnson syndrome (liver disorder)
- Rotor syndrome (liver disorder)
- Past or present stroke*
- Undiagnosed vaginal bleeding
- Undiagnosed urinary bleeding
- Missed abortion*
- Breastfeeding
  Note: Women are having babies at an older age and physicians are prescribing HRT to younger women.
- History of jaundice during pregnancy*
- Sickle-cell anemia*
- Previous or existing liver tumors*

LIST 7

Progestin pharmaceuticals: warnings and precautions

REASONS 134 THROUGH 144:

Discontinue at earliest signs of:

- Thrombotic disorders*
- Retinal thrombosis
- Eye bulging or drooping*
- Papilledema (choked eye disk)
- Unusually severe headaches
- Liver tumor*
- Jaundice*
- Hepatitis
- Pregnancy*
- Pulmonary embolism* (clot)
- Partial or complete loss of vision*
- Double vision*
- Migraine*
- Retinal vascular lesions (eye circulation)
- Gallbladder disease*
- Itching of the whole body*
- Hypertension*
- Unusual upper abdominal symptoms*

Use special monitoring in patients with:

- Preexisting fluid retention*
- Depression*
- Breakthrough bleeding*
- Epilepsy*
- Obesity*
- Sickle-cell anemia*
- Insulin and antidiabetic requirements may change*
- Adrenocorticoid function may be altered (adrenals)
- High doses may produce Cushing's disease symptoms

- Progestins slowly eliminated from body
- May mask the onset of menopause if taken by premenopausal women
- Many pathology tests may be affected, especially when estrogens are also taken. Patients may need to withdraw drug for two months and then retest.
- Follow general precautions with respect to medical checks as for estrogen: heart,* circulation,* blood,* kidney, and liver disorders.*

LIST 8

Adverse reactions: progestin pharmaceuticals

REASONS 145 THROUGH 158:

- Thrombophlebitis (vein clot/inflammation)*
- Pulmonary embolism* (lung clot or air bubble)
- Nervousness*
- Unusual fatigue*
- Drowsiness
- Headache*
- Loss of coordination
- Unwanted hair growth*
- Hair loss*
- Fever
- Liver tumors*
- Hepatitis*
- Nausea*
- Breast tenderness*
- Changes in cervical erosion
- Cushing's disease*
- Swelling of ankles and feet*
- Changes in calcium and potassium levels
- Increase in white cells and platelets
- Congenital anomalies* (if pregnant)
- Heart and brain thrombosis* (clot)

- Brain hemorrhage
- Insomnia
- Depression*
- Dizziness*
- Tremor
- Rash/itching*
- Acne*
- Sweating
- Abdominal pain*
- Jaundice*
- Gallstones*
- Appetite changes*
- Breast secretions*
- Changes in cervical/vaginal secretions
- Weight gain*
- Increase in blood pressure*
- Changes in liver enzymes*
- Shock/allergic reactions*

In *MIMS Annual* it is stated that:

- "The target group with increased risk of cardiovscular disease who would be most responsive to the treatment has not been clearly defined."
- "If a decision to use medroxyprogesterone acetate is made, patients should be encouraged to use other measures such as dietary changes, exercise, and smoking cessation."

LIST 9

Progestins

**Anomalies: problems listed in a U.S. pharmaceutical
reference text but not in Australia USPDI,**
Drug Information for the Health Care Professional, vol. I, 18th ed.,
(Rockville, Md.: U.S. Pharmacopeial Convention Inc., 1998).

REASONS 159 THROUGH 165:

- Use care in prescribing when central nervous system disorders, such as convulsions, are present.
- Some progestins, specifically androgenic progestins, might increase bad cholesterol and lower the good cholesterol.
- Dry mouth
- Unusual thirst
- Ovarian enlargement or ovarian cyst formation
- Hot flashes

LIST 10

Combination pharmaceuticals:
additional to the above-listed adverse effects

REASONS 166 THROUGH 172:

Estracombi: estrogen and progestin patches

- Uterine spasm
- Painful sex
- Risk of breast cancer probably as for estrogen
- Painful urination
- Leg pain (not thromboembolic)
- Extent of drug interactions not known

Primodian depot: synthetic estrogen plus testosterone

- Adverse reactions relating to masculinization

LIST 11

Additional adverse reactions reported in medical journals

REASONS: 173 THROUGH 193:

- Addiction potential of estrogens, especially with implants
- Alcohol plus HRT increases breast cancer risk
- Androgens plus HRT increase liver abnormalities and cancer
- Arthritis incidence increased

- Back pain increased
- Biochemistry altered; at least thirteen changes affecting other hormones, organs, and blood
- Bleeding disorders and diagnostic complications
- Breast cancer incidence understated
- Cancer incidence increased, including cervical, endometrial, ovarian, and liver cancers
- Cigarette smoking plus HRT: added effects not resolved
- Deafness cases
- Endometrial disorders widespread, plus diagnostic difficulties
- Mammographic density increases
- Muscle weakness and higher fat-to-muscle ratios
- Panic disorder cases
- Polypharmacy: one drug leads to another
- Lupus possibly increased
- Suicide and mental illness increased
- Transient ischemic attacks (circulatory blockages)

LIST 12

Other problems reported by physicians and pharmacists

REASONS 194 THROUGH 200:

- Adverse effects not theoretical; HRT abandoned by many women
  Underreporting or nonacknowledgment of adverse effects
  Patients often report that physicians tell them that a symptom is
    not a side effect of HRT when it is
- Consumer product information unreliable and biased
  Comparisons of different programs not valid
  False or premature claims, such as preventing dementia
  Estrogen's purported benefits may be offset by combining it with
    other hormones
  Prescribing practices are different between countries and physicians
    within countries.

- Costs increased due to a range of suggested monitoring while on HRT
- Dissenting doctors; increase in numbers and diverse opinions
- Environmental overflow of pharmaceutical estrogens is a possibility
- Immune system alterations and nutrient interactions are much wider than generally listed

I have not counted the following in the lists of reasons why you shouldn't take HRT because they represent a personal view, but I am sure at least some physicians would agree with them.

- Dampens body's own hormone production
- Exaggeration of potential symptoms to get women to take HRT
- False sense of security, that is, thinking HRT will prevent various problems of aging
- Inappropriate prescribing, such as to menstruating women
- Information available to physicians different to public information
- Medical studies may be short-term only or biased, for example, not looking at a range of side effects
- It is unnatural to give "young" hormones to older women.
- Safer hormones are not always prescribed.

Coming Off Hormone Replacement Therapy

*M*any women abandon hormone replacement therapy treatment because of adverse reactions or fears of increasing cancer risk. Sometimes the reason is simply because HRT does not help their symptoms. Of this group, about one-third have no problems or actually feel better without HRT, one-third experience mild flushing or other symptoms, and the rest have severe withdrawal symptoms that are often worse than when they went through natural menopause.

Women may go through a period of fairly rapid bone loss when they stop taking HRT. In other words, HRT only temporarily postpones this significant health problem, and abandoning treatment seems to create what I call a "second menopause."

Because withdrawal effects are quite common, I recommend a gradual tapering, taking approximately one month to come off the medication for every year it has been taken, unless there is an urgent reason for going cold turkey. I do not have a precise formula because it depends on the type of hormones, the dosage, and the individual, but the following is my general procedure. If you are going through a particularly stressful time, wait until things settle down before coming off HRT because the changing hormone pattern might add to your turmoil.

1. Reduce the dosage of the current prescription for a few months. Start introducing a variety of phytoestrogenic foods into the diet on a regular basis in normal dietary quantities. (These foods and other health-enhancing treatments are given in chapters 3, 4, and 5).
2. Use the lowest possible dose of external natural hormones for a further few months.
3. Reduce the pharmaceutical hormones to zero and take 500 IU (300 to 400 mg) of vitamin E twice daily and the maximum dose of Siberian ginseng. The purpose of these two remedies is to give the body support to see if it can produce enough hormones to avoid flushing and other symptoms.

Continue these remedies for the following month, while continuing to expand your phytoestrogenic diet.

Symptoms such as hot flashes tend to occur about three weeks after complete discontinuation of the hormones, but remember that some women also feel better then. I recommend a strong herbal formula if symptoms occur. A list of recommended herbs is given in chapter 5.

I encourage a lifelong use of a whole-food diet that is rich in phytoestrogens as well as postural checks and regular physical activity.

APPENDIX III

The Wild Yam (Cream) Scam

*W*ild yam external cream and wild yam sublingual drops are unproven and are highly unlikely to confer any therapeutic benefit. You're better off spending your money on organic fruits and vegetables, phytoestrogenic foods, or a multivitamin.

When these creams first came onto the market, they were promoted as having progesteronic effects in the body. When this claim was proven incorrect by various laboratory tests,[1] the manufacturers countered by saying the effect was to increase DHEA (an adrenal hormone). When this claim, too, was found to be incorrect, some manufacturers then claimed that their wild yam products were estrogenic.

Even if wild yam does have some estrogenic effect (which is unlikely in the weak products being sold over the counter and by multilevel marketing), manufacturers have yet to produce evidence that such an estrogenic effect actually occurs in the human body. Some manufacturers are now using vague terms such as "hormone balancing" and "feminizing" to promote their products.

WILD YAM AS A TRADITIONAL HERB

According to the *King's American Dispensatory*, 1898, and the *British Herbal Pharmacopoeia*, 1983, wild yam is a long-standing, traditional remedy for colic, cramps, muscle pain, and gallbladder problems. Tradition means that an herb has stood the test of time by professional herbalists and is not something that has been recently invented.

Not one early authoritative herbal book mentions wild yam for treating premenstrual syndrome, menopause, or weak bones. There is no traditional support whatsoever for wild yam's use as a hormonal remedy, nor could I find any reference for its use as a remedy applied to the skin to produce either an external or internal therapeutic effect.

Before manufacturers promote a new therapeutic indication or a new way of using an established herb, we should insist that they provide good scientific or clinical evidence that it works in the way proposed and that it has minimal adverse effects.

THE SCIENTIFIC EVIDENCE FOR WILD YAM

1. A human study showed that wild yam beneficially modifies the body's fats and functions as an antioxidant.[2] My assessment is that maximum medicinal doses would be required to make any impact on cholesterol levels.

2. An old medical report suggested that yams could be used for estrogen replacement but only if eaten in large quantities and not cooked.[3] Vegetable yams, such as those consumed in the Trobriand Islands in the Pacific, are never eaten raw and are probably not digestible in an uncooked state. Furthermore, there are over fifty-three different species of yam,[4] and what is true of one may not apply to all or any of the others. Medicinal wild yam has a shocking taste and is not eaten as a vegetable.

3. A 1967 scientific study reported that there was an extremely small amount of estrogenic biological activity in yam,[5] and the researchers stated that most, if not all, would be inactivated by

cooking[6] and presumably by processing. These very old studies may need reevaluation; the recent evidence shows that the common phytoestrogens are not damaged by heat. Diosgenin is only one of the hormone-like compounds (steroidal sapogenins) in yams. The quantity of total steroidal sapogenin content in fifty-three species of yams varied from a trace to 13 percent.[7]

4. Estrogenic action of oral diosgenin on the breast tissue of mice has been reported. The researchers reported that diosgenin showed a lack of progesterogenic action.[8] The doses given to mice in this study were the equivalent of between 24 to 48 grams daily (5 to 10 teaspoons) of the herb for a 132-pound human, assuming a 5 percent diosgenin content. These dosages are 400,000 to 800,000 times more than the theoretical diosgenin content in some U.S. internal and external wild yam products, so it is ridiculous to recommend a dose of ten drops a day (or ½ teaspoon of a weak external cream) for hormonal effects in humans. There is also some debate as to whether wild yam contains diosgenin or dioscin. Furthermore, the label on one U.S. sublingual drops product states that the amount of wild yam in the extract is 40 milligrams per milliliter, which means that only ¹⁄₂₅ of the product is the herb. The mouse study's dosage also exceeds the maximum medicinal dose used by professional herbalists, which is currently between 2 and 12 grams (½ to 2½ teaspoons daily). Thus, it is not reasonable to cite this study on mice, which used an isolated compound extracted from a yam root.

5. A double-blind placebo controlled trial has been conducted on menopausal women by Australian scientists, and the wild yam cream product was shown to be no better than placebo.[9] This finding, however, did not stop the manufacturer from subsequently promoting its product for menopausal symptoms and even suggesting that the trial showed its product to be favorable.

6. There is no clinical or scientific evidence that wild yam, either internally or externally, has any effect on reproductive hormones in humans at medicinal dosages. Because enormous doses have

shown estrogenic effects in animals and actually augment biological estrogens, however, I would not use it for women on prescribed estrogens or for women with symptoms relating to high natural estrogens, such as endometriosis.

If you have been using wild yam cream or drops, don't worry about them being harmful. The dosages are so small that it is highly improbable that the wild yam in this form has any measurable effect whatsoever. All you have lost is your money.

ETHICAL QUESTIONS

Some U.S. and Australian manufacturers have been selling wild yam herbal creams and drops, but the products actually contained progesterone hormone (and usually some of the herb as well). Progesterone can be manufactured in a laboratory from various compounds in various plants, but there is no comparison between an herb and a hormone. Because plants contain about 500 different compounds, a distinction must also be made between an herb and an isolated compound in the herb.

The Australian government made it illegal to add hormones to herbs, and all hormones are permitted by prescription only. It is not legal to spike natural remedies with hormones, nor is it safe or ethical. You may have a condition for which the hormone is contraindicated, and you have the right to know if you are taking a hormone or an herb. All medicinal hormones (irrespective of the way they are manufactured) can have adverse effects and should be prescribed only when there is a known deficiency.

At least two manufacturers' surveys showed that wild yam creams and drops are effective, yet these surveys do not actually show that the products are any better than placebo. For example, one manufacturer claims that diosgenin, when taken orally, penetrates directly into the adrenal gland. This statement is a gross misrepresentation, because the animal studies cited showed that most of the diosgenin was excreted in the feces, virtually none was absorbed, none could be detected in the serum after one large dose, and even after massive doses for four weeks only small amounts could be detected in serum.[10] The animal dose was the equivalent of giving a human 120 grams of the herb, or more than ten times the maximum medicinal dose.

According to the promotional material of the various manufacturers, wild yam cream is recommended or implied for treatment of the following:

- Menstrual symptoms
- Premenstrual syndrome
- Menopausal symptoms
- To improve energy, stamina, and endurance
- To stimulate and regulate hormones
- Fluid retention
- Bloating
- Breast swelling/fibrocystic disease
- Depression
- Low libido
- Uterine fibroids
- Weight gain
- Fat deposition at hips and thighs
- Heavy or irregular menses
- Craving for sweets
- Symptoms of low thyroid (cold hands, etc.)
- Osteoporosis
- Breast cancer
- Ovarian cancer
- Asthma
- Estrogen dominance
- Hirsutism (unwanted hair growth)
- Bladder problems

I have yet to see any evidence that it does even one of these things. Although placebo remedies such as wild yam cream may be acceptable for treating, say, premenstrual syndrome or menopausal symptoms, using it for conditions such as osteoporosis could be harmful. Instead, those women should be taking something that at least has some therapeutic potential.

The majority of wild yam creams include a varied selection of other ingredients such as herbs and oils. One manufacturer states that its brand is superior because of particular added oils, another refers to the value of homoeopathic wild yam, another states that all the added components are important, and yet another proudly promotes that its product has no other ingredients to fill up the jar or interfere with absorption. There is no evidence that a tiny dose of any external herbal cream does anything internally, although some aromatic oils and other substances may have some benefits.

Much of the promotional material refers to publications about natural hormones but fails to clarify that the product being promoted is actually an herb. My interpretation is that apparently most manufacturers of wild yam cream do not know the difference between an herb and a hormone.

HOW ARE WILD YAM CREAM DOSAGES DERIVED?

The typical recommended dose of wild yam cream is ¼ to ½ teaspoon morning and night. This dosage has been established simply by referring to the dosage of progesterone hormone cream.

Most wild yam creams contain about 10 percent of the herb or less. Plants are colored, so a white or pale cream indicates that an herbal product is weak. Start reading labels carefully, and if you need clarification, contact the manufacturer.

Assuming a 5 percent diosgenin content and a 4 percent absorption (as with hormones), the purported active component (diosgenin) in a daily dosage of cream is less than 0.5 milligram, that is, about one six-thousandth of a teaspoon! Natural progesterone creams have a dosage of 20 to 30 milligrams, which is about sixty times more than the theoretical diosgenin content of a wild yam cream dose. Furthermore, we know to a certain extent what hormones do in the human body and we know that they are absorbed across the skin, but we don't know either of these things in respect to diosgenin or wild yam.

The cost of wild yam cream has presumably been arrived at by the same copycat method. Some retail outlets are selling a 50 gram jar of wild yam cream for more than $30. The actual cost of the ingredients is only a few dollars.

WHY DO MANY WOMEN APPARENTLY FEEL BETTER FROM USING WILD YAM CREAMS AND DROPS?

The placebo response is particularly powerful for symptoms that are linked to the nervous system. Most double-blind controlled medical studies show varying percentages of response to placebos. For conditions such as premenstrual syndrome and menopausal flushing, 25 to 94 percent of women have reduced symptoms when taking placebos. Placebo remedies should be inexpensive and should not be used in situations where necessary treatment is avoided or delayed. (Better yet, use something that has at least the potential to give health benefits.)

True menopausal symptoms such as hot flashes diminish in time without any treatment. If you have to take three lots of remedies over a period of time, the last prescription is bound to be the most effective. The same principle applies to all self-limiting health problems. In other words, "tincture of time" can be an effective remedy!

Nearly all menopausal women feel better in the cooler weather. Some relapse in the hottest months of summer and their symptoms disappear by themselves in the fall. The timing of the treatment may be a significant factor.

From your own experience and from the evidence cited in chapter 10, the mind can be quite powerful. Positive thinking is an impressive and inexpensive therapy.

Wild yam is a scam for a number of reasons.

- There is a distinct difference among an herb, an isolated compound in an herb, and a hormone.
- Wild yam as an internal remedy has some proven therapeutic benefits; wild yam cream and sublingual drops have no benefits and defy common sense.
- A teaspoon of wild yam external cream or a few drops of a weak herbal extract can hardly be therapeutic for any condition, especially as a systemic (internal) treatment.

- Although we have some information on phytoestrogenic foods and herbs, we should be cautious about ascribing specific human hormonal effects resulting from topical or even oral use of herbs.
- Internally, at a proper medicinal dose, it is possible that wild yam may be estrogenic, but we do not know if that is a good or harmful hormonal effect. I do not prescribe wild yam to young women for more than a few months when treating irritable bowel syndrome and digestive problems. It may help some types of arthritis where there is muscle spasm. Wild yam as an internal herbal remedy has rational uses including improving bile flow and treating colic.

I have spent twenty years researching plant hormones and am very disappointed that products such as wild yam cream and very diluted liquid extracts downgrade natural therapies. Nowadays there are thousands of good studies to support effective natural products.

Because wild yam cream and drops have no tradition, no scientific support, no reasonable clinical evidence, and do not conform to common sense, don't believe the unbelievable. Use your own common sense.

Case Studies of Osteoporosis

*S*ome governments now recommend that two years is the preferred time before a bone mineral density scan is repeated to evaluate the effectiveness of a program. If possible, I aim for a one-year test to evaluate if the program is successful.

PATIENT NO. 1 (MYSELF)

At fifty-nine years of age, I had considered myself healthy and fit, apart from recurring troublesome arthritis. For about twenty years I had been mainly vegetarian (with occasional lapses) and had exercised regularly.

I had a varied diet, mainly vegetables, legumes, whole grains, dairy and soy products, eggs, nuts, fruits, and occasionally fish and the odd treat. I had no cigarettes, virtually no alcohol, no added salt, two cups of weak coffee a day, and no supplements except for fairly regular herbal tonics and intermittent natural remedies for arthritis.

My weekly exercise routine included between four to seven hours of moderate yoga stretching and strengthening exercises; about sixty minutes jogging; and eight hours of light to moderate physical work, such as gardening, walking, and sometimes swimming. Arthritic pain sometimes interrupted this program.

You can imagine my disappointment to discover that, according to a bone density scan, I had moderate osteoporosis in the upper femur and lumbar spine. Why were my bones in such a state? I have hundreds of relatives, most of whom lead very unhealthy lifestyles, yet to my knowledge none had sustained an osteoporotic fracture despite many of them living normal lifespans. Perhaps my bone mineral content had been low since childhood due to a very high intake of cow's milk along with fairly high meat, high fat, and sugar. When I was at school, all students had a compulsory half-pint bottle of milk to drink for both morning and afternoon tea. Maybe I had lost too much weight in my forties when I became a vegetarian. Was my adult calcium intake too low, was my diet somewhat deficient in some nutrient, or was there something wrong with my bone collagen? Would my bones have been worse had I not had those twenty relatively healthy years? Or, was I one of those few low-risk people who simply end up on the wrong side of the statistical chart?

At the time, my local physician pressured me to take HRT, but I resisted and kept up my current lifestyle, making a conscious decision not to avoid accidents. About a year after my first scan, when I was clearing the leaves from my roof gutters, I fell about 14 feet onto the concrete path below, landing on one leg before falling to the ground. Amazingly, no bones were broken. Up to that time I had also worked as a horticulturist one day a week and had often carried bags of sand that weighed more than my own body weight. I also did some minor rock climbing and had a few falls over the years. Because I was around the fracture threshold, why were no bones broken from various serious falls and other hazards when some people sustain a fracture getting out of a chair? Perhaps it was luck, relatively strong muscles, flexible joints, or flexible bone matrix. After all, the minerals are laid down into the bone collagen.

Subsequently, I thought I should not rely on luck. Because my diet and lifestyle were seemingly healthy, the best option was judged to be a supplement program. My recommended program is given below.

Recommended Program

Dietary Advice   Increase fish intake. Diet was possibly low in protein. Increase nuts, seeds, avocado, and quality oils, such as virgin olive oil. Current diet too low in fats.

Supplements

- Osteoapatite with boron (a form of calcium plus other nutrients)
  2 tablets after breakfast, 2 tablets before bed (in ½ glass soy milk)
  Contents: Microcrystalline hydroxyapatite 460 milligrams (115 milligrams elemental calcium), vitamin D_3 (cholecalciferol) 50 IU (1.25 µg), manganese 5 milligrams, zinc 3 milligrams, copper 300 micrograms , boron 1 milligram (elemental levels).
- Collagenics
  1 tablet after breakfast, 1 tablet before bed
  Contents: Horsetail herb, proline, lysine, cystine, vitamin C, magnesium, manganese, glutamine, xylose, iron, vitamin B_6, vitamin B_5.
- Vitamin E, 500 IU (335 mg) water-soluble form
  1 capsule after breakfast
  (Diet for past ten years assessed to be low in vitamin E.)
- Magnesium
  1 tablet after breakfast, 1 tablet before bed
  Contents: Elemental magnesium 46 milligrams, plus a little potassium and calcium (orotates and aspartates).

Aim   To improve the nutrients (in addition to calcium) assessed to be somewhat deficient in this patient's diet.

Result of One-Year Program   No weight change occurred.
   Compliance with the program was about 75 percent; sometimes only half the daily dose was taken.

	Beginning (g/cm^2)	End (g/cm^2)	Improvement %
Lumbar 2–4 (lower back)	0.86	0.92	7
Femoral neck (upper leg)	0.77	0.87	13

An average of 10 percent increase in one year is considered significant (excellent).

As the bone mineral density "normalized," half the dose was suggested as a long-term maintenance program.

Interpretation of Results   Nutritional supplements can increase bone mineral density if you are marginally deficient in nutrients.

PATIENTS 2 AND 3

Two women with mild osteoporosis, both in their mid-fifties, better than average diet (high vegetables, fruits, whole grains, semivegetarian, a little fish and occasional meat), no major dietary or lifestyle excesses, both walking about two hours per week and reasonably active. Both natural therapy adherents. Not taking HRT, pharmaceuticals, or supplements, other than B vitamins and vitamin C.

Recommended program

A diet high in phytoestrogens, along the lines given in chapter 3, plus 1 more hour exercise per week, either at a fitness center or more walking.

Aim   To evaluate the long-term effectiveness of dietary and exercise improvements as a means of increasing bone mineral density.

Result of One-Year Program
No significant weight change.
Compliance estimated at 80 percent.

One patient stayed the same, the other lost 3 percent (average of femoral neck and lumbar spine).
Both reported feeling better and surprised at the poor result.

Interpretation of Results   If you are already eating healthily and exercising reasonably, improvements in these areas are probably unlikely to bring about an improvement in bone mineral density.

PATIENT NO. 4

A fifty-seven-year-old woman who had been on HRT for eight years but who wanted to come off because she had a family history of breast cancer and was beginning to put on weight. Her diet was marginally better than a typical diet, and she walked regularly but not vigorously. She had a full-time job.

Recommended Program

Dietary and Lifestyle Advice
Phytoestrogen diet, at least one serving daily.
Reduce meat, aim to have two vegetarian meals per week.

Supplements
Same as Patient No. 1, but magnesium was omitted.
Instead of osteoapatite with boron, she took a plain hydroxyapatite, each tablet containing 240 milligrams elemental calcium.
Dose: 1 tablet of each after breakfast and again before bed.

Aim   To evaluate a moderate, mixed program on a patient with mild osteoporosis.

Result of One-Year Program
Weight loss of 10 pounds.
Compliance around 90 percent.

	Beginning (g/cm²)	End (g/cm²)	Improvement %
L2–L4	0.91	0.93	2
Femoral neck	0.79	0.81	2

Interpretation of Results   Disappointing at first glance but because she had been on HRT from the time of menopause, she may have experienced what I call "second menopause" when coming off the hormones, that is, a year or so of very rapid bone loss. The program may have actually offset a substantial loss. Would boron and magnesium supplementation have made any difference? Was her weight loss linked to the somewhat disappointing result?

PATIENT NO. 5

A forty-nine-year-old yoga teacher, recently stopped menstruating, twenty years vegetarian, yogic lifestyle, some joint and muscle pain, previous history of absence of periods for four years (amenorrhea), currently mild osteoporosis.

Recommended Program

Diet and Lifestyle   Eat fresh fish three times weekly; brisk walking thirty minutes every second day in addition to yoga. The patient's diet was good but possibly a little low in protein.

Supplements

- Calcium citrate formula
    Contents: Calcium citrate 250 milligrams elemental, hydroxyapatite 115 milligrams, plus magnesium, zinc, manganese, silica, vitamin D, and Vitamin K.
- Fish oil combination (enteric coated product)
    Contents 500 milligrams salmon oil, equivalent to 90 milligrams eicosapentaenoic acid and 60 milligrams docosahexaenoic acid, evening primrose oil equivalent to 50 milligrams gamma-linolenic acid, vitamin E 34 milligrams (50 IU).

- Boron and magnesium: 3 milligrams boron, 124 milligrams magnesium (elemental levels)

    Dose of one tablet of each before breakfast and again before bed.

Aim   To prevent the substantial bone mineral loss that commonly occurs immediately following menopause.

Result of One-Year Program   Compliance with supplements about 90 percent, diet and lifestyle 30 percent compliance due to changing jobs, residence.

	Beginning (g/cm^2)	End (g/cm_2)	Improvement %
L2–L4	0.91	0.90	no change
Femoral neck	0.89	0.89	no change

Interpretation of Results   Similar to previous case, indicating that it may be possible to avoid the sudden mineral loss following the cessation of periods. Patient was keen to see if a different program and more adherence to diet and lifestyle could improve her bones.

Following Year

Supplements Prescribed   Hydroxyapatite, a collagen supplement and the fish oil combination; all twice daily. A multivitamin/mineral was to be taken once daily if the diet was not followed reasonably. Phytoestrogenic foods were to be used more generously; food combining to get complete protein; some seaweeds and whey powder added to cereals; and herbal vinegar added to salads, vegetables, and the main meal to help with digestion and absorption. The patient also started some physical workouts with weights.

After one year on this program, her lumbar spine (L2–L4) increased by 2 percent and the femoral neck 7 percent. The patient now has a femoral neck reading better than average and her spine is slightly less than average, so there is no need for other than minimal supplementation and adherence to diet and lifestyle.

The above examples are but a few cases from my patients' records. Overall, the results of over thirty patients have resulted in an average annual increase of 5 percent in bone mineral density. About 20 percent of cases showed slight decreases (most occurring in patients who have recently stopped menstruating), 15 percent show excellent increases, and the majority show no change or a modest increase.

I consider no change a satisfactory result if occurring one to two years immediately following menopause or one to two years immediately following cessation of HRT because that is when major bone mineral losses may occur. For other women I expect at least a small increase in bone mineral density levels.

Overall, the best results occur with a calcium citrate combination, a fish oil combination, boron and magnesium, and a collagen remedy. I now advise all patients to exercise in line with chapter 7 and to eat a varied diet rich in phytoestrogens.

There is no guarantee that any pharmaceutical or natural program will improve your bones, but I recommend trying a natural therapy program because it has beneficial side effects compared with the adverse reactions of pharmaceuticals. Most of my osteoporotic patients have reported significant reductions in joint problems and arthritis while on the program.

Notes

Chapter 1

1. M. Hunter, "The South-East England Longitudinal Study of the Climacteric and Postmenopause," *Maturitas* 14 (1992): 117–26.
2. Australian Department of Community Services and Health, *National Women's Health Policy* (Canberra: Australian Government Printing Service, 1989).
3. N. Notelovitz and P. Van Keep (eds.), *The Climacteric in Perspective* (Boston: MTP Press, 1986).
4. N. J. Kenney et al., (eds.), *The Complexities of Women* (Dubuque, Iowa: Kendall/Hunt, 1992).
5. K. A. Matthews et al., "Influences of Natural Menopause on Psychological Characteristics and Symptoms of Middle-Aged Healthy Women," *Journal of Consulting and Clinical Psychology* 58 (1990): 345–51.
6. J. G. Green, "The Cross-Sectional Legacy: An Introduction to Longitudinal Studies of the Climacteric," *Maturitas* 14 (1992): 95–101.
7. N. Notelovitz and P. Van Keep (eds.), *The Climacteric in Perspective* (Boston: MTP Press, 1986).

8. H. Shimizu et al., "Serum Oestrogen Levels in Postmenopausal Women: Comparison of American Whites and Japanese in Japan," *British Journal of Cancer* 62 (1990): 451–53.

Chapter 2

1. B. R. Carr, "HRT Management: The American Experience," *European Journal of Obstetrics, Gynecology, and Reproductive Biology* 64, Suppl. (1996): S17–20.
2. M. W. DeGregorio and T. L. Taras, "Hormone Replacement Therapy and Breast Cancer: Revisiting the Issues," *Journal of the American Pharmacy Association Washington* 38 (1998): 738–44.
3. J. C. Montgomery et al., "Effect of Oestrogen and Testosterone Implants on Psychological Disorders in the Climacteric," *The Lancet* I (1987): 297–99.
4. S. Bewley and T. H. Bewley, "Drug Dependence with Estrogen Replacement Therapy," *The Lancet* 339 (1992): 290–91.
5. E. S. Ginsburg et al., "Effects of Alcohol Ingestion on Estrogens in Postmenopausal Women," *Journal of the American Medical Association* 276 (1996): 1747–51.
6. S. P. Dourakis and G. Tolis, "Sex Hormonal Preparations and the Liver," *European Journal of Contraception and Reproductive Health Care* 3 (1998): 7–16.
7. E. C. G. Grant, E. H. Price, and C. M. Steel, "Risks of Hormone Replacement Therapy," *The Lancet* 354 (1999): 1302–3.
8. E. Arteaga et al., "In Vitro Effect of Estradiol, Progesterone, and Testosterone on LDL-Cholesterol Oxidation in Postmenopausal Women" (paper presented at the Eighth International Congress on the Menopause, Sydney, 3–7 November 1996).
9. K. Wilkins, "Hormone Replacement Therapy and Incident Arthritis," *Health Reports* 11 (1999): 49–57.
10. E. M. Dennison et al., "Hormone Replacement Therapy, Other Reproductive Variables, and Symptomatic Hip Osteoarthritis in Elderly White Women: A Case-Control Study," *British Journal of Rheumatology* 37 (1998): 1198–202.

11. R. J. Troisi et al., "Evidence for an Estrogen Contribution to the Pathogenesis of Adult-Onset Asthma," *American Journal of Epidemiology* 139 (1994): S21.

12. J. O. Bryndildsen and M. L. Hammar, "Is Hormone Replacement Therapy a Risk Factor for Low Back Pain Among Postmenopausal Women?" (paper presented at the Eighth International Congress on the Menopause, Sydney, 3–7 November 1996).

13. E. C. G. Grant, *Sexual Chemistry* (London: Cedar, 1994).

14. U. H. Winkler, "Effects of Androgens on Hemostasis," *Maturitas* 24 (1996): 147–55.

15. B. J. Orr-Walker et al., "Hormone Replacement Therapy Causes Respiratory Alkalosis in Normal Postmenopausal Women," *Journal of Clinical Endocrinology and Metabolism* 84 (1999): 1997–2001.

16. F. Nagele et al., "Hysteroscopy in Women with Abnormal Uterine Bleeding on Hormone Replacement Therapy: A Comparison with Postmenopausal Bleeding," *Fertility and Sterility* 65 (1996): 1145–50.

17. A. A. Akkad et al., "Abnormal Iterine Bleeding on Hormone Replacement: The Importance of Intrauterine Structural Abnormalities," *Obstetrics and Gynecology* 86 (1995): 330–34.

18. Collaborative Group on Hormonal Factors in Breast Cancer, "Breast Cancer and Hormone Replacement Therapy," *The Lancet* 350 (1997): 1047–59.

19. V. Beral et al., "Use of HRT and the Subsequent Risk of Cancer," *Journal of Epidemiology and Biostatistics* 4 (1999): 191–210.

20. L. J. Hofseth et al., "Hormone Replacement Therapy with Estrogen or Estrogen Plus Medroxyprogesterone Acetate Is Associated with Increased Epithelial Proliferation in the Normal Postmenopausal Breast," *Journal of Clinical Endocrinology and Metabolism* 84 (1999): 4559–65.

21. B. S. Hulka, "Hormone Replacement Therapy (HRT) and Breast Cancer" (paper presented at the Eighth International Congress on the Menopause, Sydney, 3–7 November 1996).

22. B. Rockhill, G. A. Colditz, and B. Rosner, "Bias in Breast Cancer Analyses Due to Error in Age at Menopause," *American Journal of Epidemiology* 151 (2000): 404–8.

23. B. Fowble et al., "Postmenopausal Hormone Replacement Therapy: Effect on Diagnosis and Outcome in Early Stage Invasive Breast Cancer Treated with Conservative Surgery and Radiation," *Journal of Clinical Oncology* 17 (1999): 1680–88.

24. I. Persson, E. Thurfjell, and L. Holmberg, "Effect of Estrogen and Estrogen-Progestin Replacement Regimens on Mammographic Breast Parenchymal Density," *Journal of Clinical Oncology* 15 (1997): 3201–7.

25. P. E. Belchetz, "Hormonal Treatment of Postmenopausal Women," *New England Journal of Medicine* 330 (1994): 1062–71.

26. J. Eden, "Should Women Who Have Had Breast Cancer Take Hormone Replacement Therapy?" *Maturitas* 22 (1995): 69–70.

27. E. C. G. Grant et al., "Breast Cancer and Hormone Exposure," *The Lancet* 348 (1996): 682.

28. J. O. White et al., "The Human Squamous Cervical Carcinoma Cell Line, HOG-1, Is Responsive to Steroid Hormones," *International Journal of Cancer* 52 (1992) 247–51.

29. S. Duun, K. Roed-Petersen, and J. W. Michelsen, "Endometrioid Carcinoma Arising from Endometriosis of the Sigmoid Colon During Estrogenic Treatment," *Acta Obstetricia et Gynecologica Scandinavica* 72 (1993): 676–78.

30. M. A. Habiba, S. C. Bell, and F. Al-Azzawi, "Endometrial Responses to Hormone Replacement Therapy: Histological Features Compared with Those of Late Luteal Phase Endometrium," *Human Reproduction* 13 (1998): 1674–82.

31. C. Rodriquez et al., "Estrogen Replacement Therapy and Fatal Ovarian Cancer," *American Journal of Epidemiology* 141 (1995): 828–35.

32. P. P. Garg et al., "Hormone Replacement Therapy and the Risk of Epithelial Ovarian Carcinoma: A Meta-Analysis," *Obstetrics and Gynecology* 92 (1998): 472–79.

33. E. Negri et al., "Hormonal Therapy for Menopause and Ovarian Cancer in a Collaborative Re-Analysis of European Studies," *International Journal of Cancer* 80 (1999): 848–51.

34. H. P. Schneider, "HRT and Cancer Risk: Separating Fact from Fiction," *Maturitas* 33, Suppl. (1999): S65–72.

35. T. W. Meade and M. R. Vickers, "HRT and Cardiovascular Disease," *Journal of Epidemiology and Biostatistics* 4 (1999): 165–90.
36. S. C. MacLennan, A. H. MacLennan, and P. Ryan, "Colorectal Cancer and Estrogen Replacement Therapy: A Meta-Analysis of Epidemiological Studies," *Medical Journal of Australia* 162 (1995): 491–93.
37. C. M. Beale and P. Collins, "The Menopause and the Cardiovascular System," *Baillieres Clinical Obstetrics and Gynaecology* 10 (1996): 483–513.
38. L. H. Kuller, J. A. Cauley L. Lucas et al., "Sex Steroid Hormones, Bone Mineral Density, and Risk of Breast Cancer," *Environmental Health Perspectives* 105, Suppl. (1997): S593–99.
39. E. Hogervorst et al., "The Effect of Hormone Replacement Therapy on Cognitive Function in Elderly Women," *Psychoneurendocrinology* 24 (1999): 43–68.
40. V. Beral et al., "Use of HRT and the Subsequent Risk of Cancer," *Journal of Epidemiology and Biostatistics* 4 (1999): 191–210.
41. H. P. Schneider, "Cross National Study of Women's Use of Hormone Replacement Therapy (HRT) in Europe," *International Journal of Fertility and Women's Medicine* 42 (1997): 365–75.
42. P. C. Hannaford, "Is There Sufficient Evidence for Us to Encourage the Widespread Use of Hormone Replacement Therapy to Prevent Disease?" *British Journal of General Practice* 48 (1998): 952–53.
43. J. L. Exline, I. A. Siegler, and L. A. Bastion, "Differences in Providers' Beliefs about Benefits and Risks of Hormone Replacement Therapy in Managed Care," *Journal of Women's Health* 7 (1998): 879–84.
44. E. C. G. Grant et al., "Breast Cancer and Hormone Exposure," *The Lancet* 348 (1996): 682.
45. H. P. Schneider and J. C. Gallagher, "Moderation of the Daily Dose of HRT: Benefits for Patients," *Maturitas* 33, Suppl. (1999): S25–9.
46. K. Laine et al., "Plasma Tacrine Concentrations Are Significantly Increased by Concomitant Hormone Replacement Therapy," *Clinical Pharmacology and Therapeutics* 66 (1999): 602–8.
47. W. Schubert et al., "Inhibition of 17 Beta-Estradiol Metabolism by Grapefruit Juice in Ovariectomized Women," *Maturitas* 20 (1994): 155–63.

48. R. Hart and A. Magos, "How Long Should a Woman take HRT?" *The Practitioner* 242 (1998): 114–19.
49. D. R. Halbert et al., "Hormone Replacement Therapy Usage: A 10 Year Experience of a Solo Practitioner," *Maturitas* 29 (1998): 67–73.
50. S. Kaba, T. Aoki, and T. Fukatsu, "Endometrial Cytology in Post-menopausal Hormone Replacement Therapy," *Diagnostic Cytopathology* 19 (1998): 161–67.
51. H. Maia et al., "Management of Endometrial Polyps in Menopause Patients under HRT" (paper presented at Eighth International Congress on the Menopause, Sydney, 3–7 November 1996).
52. F. I. Chinegwundoh et al., "Renal and Diaphragmatic Endometriosis De Novo Associated with Hormone Replacement Therapy," *Journal of Urology* 153 (1995): 380–81.
53. S. C. Bell et al., "Estrogen Receptor and Heat Shock Protein 27 Expression During the Late 'Pseudo-Luteal' Phase of a HRT Regimen: Adequate Estrogenic Priming" (paper presented at the Eighth International Congress on the Menopause, Sydney, 3–7 November 1996).
54. A. M. Anderson and N. E. Skakkebaek, "Exposure to Exogenous Estrogens in Food: Possible Impact on Human Development and Health," *European Journal of Endocrinology* 140 (1999): 477–85.
55. C. L. Harden et al., "The Effect of Menopause and Perimenopause on the Course of Epilepsy," *Epilepsia* 40 (1999): 1402–7.
56. T. Hachiya and N. Wake, "Breast and Thyroid Disease Screening for Perimenopausal Women by Ultrasound" (paper presented at the Eighth Congress on the Menopause, Sydney, 3–7 November 1996).
57. S. Hulley et al., "Randomized Trial of Estrogen Plus Progestin for Secondary Prevention of Coronary Heart Disease in Postmenopausal Women," *Journal of the American Medical Association* 280 (1998): 605–13.
58. E. Barrett-Connor, "Hormones and Heart Disease and Women" (paper presented at the Eighth International Congress on the Menopause, Sydney 3–7 November 1996).
59. E. Farish et al., "Effects of Tibolone Compared with a Cyclical Estrogen/Progestin Regimen on Lipoproteins" (paper presented at the

Eighth International Congress on the Menopause, Sydney, 3–7 November 1996).

60. B. L. Haddock et al., "Cardiorespiratory Fitness and Cardiovascular Disease Risk Factors in Postmenopausal Women," *Medicine and Science in Sports and Exercise* 30 (1998): 893–98.

61. M. Larkin, "Value of HRT in Women with Heart Disease Doubted," *The Lancet* 352 (1998): 627.

62. P. August and S. Oparil, "Hypertension in Women," *Journal of Clinical Endocrinology and Metabolism* 84 (1999): 1862–66.

63. R. Brunelli et al., "Hormone Replacement Therapy Affects Various Immune Cell Subsets and Natural Cytotoxicity," *Gynecologic and Obstetric Investigation* 41 (1996): 128–31.

64. B. Larson, A. Collins, and B. M. Landgren, "Urogenital and Vasomotor Symptoms in Relation to Menopausal Status and the Use of Hormone Replacement Therapy in Healthy Women During Transition to Menopause," *Maturitas* 28 (1997): 99–105.

65. A. E. Gebbie, A. Glasier, and V. Sweeting, "Incidence of Ovulation in Perimenopausal Women Before and During Hormone Replacement Therapy," *Contraception* 52 (1995): 52–54.

66. H. R. Shibata, "Hormone Replacement Therapy: Boon or Bane?" *Canadian Journal of Surgery* 38 (1995): 409–14.

67. F. P. Dunne, "Should Women with Diabetes Mellitus Receive Hormone Replacement Therapy?" *International Journal of Clinical Practice* 51 (1997): 299–303.

68. M. M. McNicholas et al., "Pain and Increased Mammographic Density in Women Receiving Hormone Replacement Therapy: A Prospective Study," *American Journal of Roentgenology* 163 (1994): 311–15.

69. A. M. Kavanagh, H. Mitchell, and G. G. Giles, "Hormone Replacement Therapy and Accuracy of Mammographic Screening," *The Lancet* 355 (2000): 270–74.

70. The Writing Group for the PEPI Trial, "Effects of Estrogen or Estrogen/Progestin Regimens on Heart Disease Risk Factors in Postmenopausal Women," *Journal of the American Medical Association* 273 (1995): 199–208.

71. E. Darj et al., "Liver Metabolism During Treatment with Estradiol and Natural Progesterone," *Gynecological Endocrinology* 7 (1993): 111−14.

72. G. Greer, *The Change* (London: Hamish Hamilton, 1991).

73. A. Collins and B. M. Landgren, "Psychosocial Factors Associated with the Use of Hormonal Replacement Therapy in a Longitudinal Follow Up of Swedish Women," *Maturitas* 28 (1997): 1−9.

74. A. J. Weisserger, K. K. Ho, and L. Lazarus, "Contrasting Effects of Oral and Transdermal Routes of Estrogen Replacement Therapy on 24-Hour Growth Hormone (GH) Secretion, Insulin-Like Growth Factor I, and GH-Binding Protein in Postmenopausal Women," *Journal of Clinical Endocrinology and Metabolism* 72 (1991): 374−81.

75. B. E. Reubinoff et al., "Effects of Hormone Replacement Therapy on Weight, Body Composition, Fat Distribution, and Food Intake in Early Postmenopausal Women: A Prospective Study," *Fertility and Sterility* 64 (1996): 963−68.

76. P. E. Belchetz, "Hormonal Treatment of Postmenopausal Women," *New England Journal of Medicine* 330 (1994): 1062−71.

77. D. M. Gruber et al., "Endometrial Cancer after Combined Hormone Replacement Therapy," *Maturitas* 31 (1999): 237−40.

78. P. E. Belchetz, "Hormonal Treatment of Postmenopausal Women," *New England Journal of Medicine* 330 (1994): 1062−71.

79. D. L. Faulkner et al., "Patient Noncompliance with Hormone Replacement Therapy: A Nationwide Estimate Using a Large Prescription Claims Database," *Menopause* 5 (1998): 226−29.

80. E. Grant, *Sexual Chemistry* (London: Cedar, 1994).

81. D. T. Felson et al., "The Effect of Postmenopausal Estrogen Therapy on Bone Mineral Density in Elderly Women," *New England Journal of Medicine* 329 (1993): 1141−46.

82. C. Christiansen et al., "Bone Mass in Postmenopausal Women after Withdrawal of Estrogen/Gestagen Replacement Therapy," *The Lancet* 1 (1981): 459−61.

83. J. McLaren-Howard, E. C. G. Grant, and S. Davies, "Hormone Replacement Therapy and Osteoporosis: Bone Enzymes and Nutrient

Imbalances," *Journal of Nutritional and Environmental Medicine* 8 (1998): 129–38.

84. M. H. Komulainen et al., "HRT and Vitamin D in Prevention of Non-Vertebral Fractures in Postmenopausal Women: A 5 Year Randomized Trial," *Maturitas* 31 (1998): 45–54.

85. J. A. Kanis, "Estrogens, the Menopause, and Osteoporosis," *Bone* 19, Suppl. (1996): S185–190.

86. T. Cundy et al., "Bone Density in Women Receiving Depot Medroxyprogesterone Acetate for Contraception," *British Medical Journal* 303 (1991): 13–16.

87. C. Paul et al., "Depot Medroxyprogesterone (Depo-Provera) and Risk of Breast Cancer," *British Medical Journal* 299 (1989): 759–62.

88. L. Dennerstein et al., "Sexuality, Hormones, and the Menopausal Transition" (paper presented at the Eighth International Congress on the Menopause," Sydney, 3–7 November 1996).

89. M. Stomati et al., "Endocrine, Neuroendocrine, and Behavioral Effects of Oral Delydroepiandrosterone Sulfate Supplementation in Postmenopausal Women," *Gynecology and Endocrinology* 13 (1999): 15–25.

90. M. L. Dembert, M. P. Dinneen, and M. S. Opsahl, "Estrogen-Induced Panic Disorder," *American Journal of Psychiatry* 151 (1994): 1246.

91. B. G. Saver, T. R. Taylor, and N. F. Woods, "Use of Hormone Replacement Therapy in Washington State: Is Prevention Being Put into Practice?" *Journal of Family Practice* 48 (1999): 364–71.

92. C. Magnusson et al., "Breast Cancer Risk Following Long-Term Estrogen and Progestin Replacement Therapy," *International Journal of Cancer* 81 (1999): 339–144.

93. J. H. Schram et al., "Influence of Two Hormone Replacement Therapy Regimens, Oral Estradiol Valerate, and Cyproterone Acetate Versus Transdermal Estradiol and Oral Dydrogesterone on Lipid Metabolism," *Maturitas* 22 (1995): 121–30.

94. W. M. Van Baal et al., "Short-Term Hormone Replacement Therapy: Reduced Plasma Levels of Soluble Adhesion Molecules," *European Journal of Clinical Investigation* 29 (1999): 913–21.

95. J. T. Comerci et al., "Continuous Low Dose Combined Hormone Replacement Therapy and the Risk of Endometrial Cancer," *Gynecologic Oncology* 64 (1997): 425–30.

96. R. N. Smith, E. F. Holland, and J. W. Studd, "The Symptomatology of Progestogen Intolerance," *Maturitas* 18 (1994): 87–91.

97. G. M. C. Rosano et al., "Medroxyprogesterone Acetate (MPA) but Not Natural Progesterone Reverses the Effect of Estradiol 17B upon Exercise Induced Myocardial Ischemia: A Double Blind Cross-Over Study" (paper presented at the Eighth International Congress on the Menopause, Sydney, 3–7 November 1996).

98. E. Darj et al., "Liver Metabolism During Treatment with Estradiol and Natural Progesterone," *Gynecologic Endocrinology* 7 (1993): 111–14.

99. J. Anasti, "Poster Session on Progesterone Cream and Postmenopausal Vasomotor Symptoms" (poster presented at the Sixteenth World Congress on Fertility and Sterility, American Society for Reproductive Medicine, 1998).

100. E. Suvanto-Luukkonen, H. Malinen, H. Sundstrom et al., "Endometrial Morphology During Hormone Replacement Therapy with Estradiol Gel Combined to Levonorgestrel-Releasing Intrauterine Device or Natural Progesterone," *Acta Obstetrica et Gynecologica Scandinavica* 77 (1998): 758–63.

101. J. R. Lee, *What Your Doctor May Not Tell You About Menopause* (New York: Warner Books, 1996, p. 167).

102. P. E. Belchez, "Hormonal Treatment of Postmenopausal Women," *New England Journal of Medicine* 330 (1994): 1062–69.

103. E. M. Alder, "Hormone Replacement Therapy and Psychological Symptoms: A Comparison of Tibolone and Conjugated Estrogens" (paper presented at the Eighth International Congress on the Menopause, Sydney, 3–7 November 1996).

104. L. Dennerstein, A. M. Smith and C. Morse, "Psychological Well-Being, Mid-Life, and the Menopause," *Maturitas* 20 (1994): 1–11.

105. M. S. Hunter and K. L. Liao, "Intentions to Use Hormone Replacement Therapy in a Community Sample of 45-Year Old Women," *Maturitas* 20 (1994): 13–23.

106. K. Takahashi et al., "Safety and Efficacy of Estriol for Symptoms of Natural or Surgically Induced Menopause," *Human Reproduction* 15 (2000): 1028–36.

107. J. Sanchez-Guerrero et al., "Postmenopausal Estrogen Therapy and the Risk for Developing Systemic Lupus Erythematosus," *Annals of Internal Medicine* 122 (1995): 430–33.

108. M. L. Slattery et al., "Hormone Replacement Therapy and Improved Survival among Postmenopausal Women Diagnosed with Colon Cancer (USA)," *Cancer Causes and Control* 10 (1999): 467–73.

109. M. M. Fung, E. Barrett-Connor, and R. R. Bettencourt, "Hormone Replacement Therapy and Stroke Risk in Older Women," *Journal of Women's Health* 8 (1999): 359–64.

110. F. Grodstein et al., "Postmenopausal Estrogen and Progestin Use and the Risk of Cardiovascular Disease," *New England Journal of Medicine* 335 (1996): 453–61.

111. E. H. Price, "Increased Risk of Mental Illness and Suicide in Oral Contraceptive and Hormone Replacement Therapy Studies," *Journal of Nutritional and Environmental Medicine* 8 (1998): 121–27.

112. D. R. Phillips, "Endometrial Ablation for Postmenopsusal Uterine Bleeding Induced by Hormone Replacement Therapy," *Journal of the American Association of Gynecologic Laparoscopists* 2 (1995): 389–93.

113. E. M. Alder, "Estradiol Implants, Patches, and Reported Symptoms" (paper presented at the Eighth International Congress on the Menopause, Sydney, 3–7 November 1996).

114. J. K. Waselenko, M. C. Nace, and B. Alving, "Women with Thrombophilia: Assessing the Risks for Thrombosis with Oral Contraceptives or Hormone Replacement Therapy," *Seminars in Thrombosis and Hemostasis* 24, Suppl. (1998): 33–39.

115. M. S. Seelig, "Interrelationship of Magnesium and Estrogen in Cardiovascular and Bone Disorders, Eclampsia, Migraine, and Premenstrual Syndrome," *Journal of the American College of Nutrition* 12 (1993): 442–58.

116. R. Strachan, D. Hughes, and R. Cowie, "Thrombosis of the Straight Sinus Complicating Hormone Replacement Therapy," *British Journal of Neurosurgery* 9 (1995): 805–8.

117. D. Strachan, "Sudden Sensorineural Deafness and Hormone Replacement Therapy," *Journal of Laryngology and Otology* 110 (1996): 1148–50.

118. I. D. Orlander et al., "Urinary Tract Infections and Estrogen Use in Older Women," *Journal of American Geriatric Society* 40 (1992): 817–20.

119. A. M. Heikkinen et al., "Long-Term Vitamin D_3 Supplementation May Have Adverse Effects on Serum Lipids during Postmenopausal Hormone Replacement Therapy," *European Journal of Endocrinology* 137 (1997): 495–502.

120. M. Herzberg et al., "The Effect of Estrogen Replacement Therapy on Zinc in Serum and Bone," *Obstetrics and Gynecology* 87 (1996): 1035–40.

121. E. Grant, *Sexual Chemistry* (London: Cedar, 1994).

122. G. Tang, P. Yip, and B. Li, "Menopausal Symptoms and General Well-Being: The Effect of Hormone Replacement Therapy in Two Groups of Chinese Women" (paper presented at the Eighth International Congress on the Menopause, Sydney, 3–7 November 1996).

Chapter 3

1. C. Nagata et al., "Effect of Soymilk Consumption on Serum Estrogen Concentrations in Premenopsusal Japanese Women," *Journal of the National Cancer Institute* 90 (1998) 1830–35.

2. A. L. Murkies et al., "Dietary Flour Supplementation Decreases Postmenopausal Hot Flushes: Effect of Soy and Wheat," *Maturitas* 21 (1995): 189–95.

3. F. S. Dalais et al., "Effects of Dietary Phytoestrogens in Postmenopausal Women," *Climacteric* 1 (1998): 124–29.

4. J. W. Erdman, "Short-Term Effects of Soybean Isoflavones on Bone in Postmenopausal Women" (paper presented at the Second International Symposium on the Role of Soy in Preventing and Treating Chronic Disease, Brussels, 15–18 September 1996).

5. S. M. Potter, "Soy Protein and Cardiovascular Disease: The Impact of Bioactive Components of Soy," *Nutrition Reviews* 56 (1998): 231–35.

6. P. J. Nestel et al., "Isoflavones from Red Clover Improve Systemic Arterial Compliance but Not Plasma Lipids in Menopausal Women," *Journal of Clinical Endocrinology and Metabolism* 84 (1999): 895–98.

7. A. Harper et al., "Antioxidant Effects of Isoflavonoids and Lignans, and Protection Against DNA Oxidation," *Free Radical Research* 31 (1999): 149–60.

8. S. Seely, "Diet and Cerebrovascular Disease," *Nutrition and Health* 2 (1983): 173–79.

9. H. Aldercreutz, "Phytoestrogens: Epidemiology and a Possible Role in Cancer Protection," *Environmental Health Perspectives* 103, Suppl. (1995): 103–12.

10. D. Ingram et al., "Case-Control Study of Phytoestrogens and Breast Cancer," *The Lancet* 350 (1997): 990–94.

11. S. Holt, *Soya for Health* (Larchmont, N.Y.: Mary Ann Liebert, Inc., 1996).

12. Consensus Opinion of the North American Menopause Society, "The Role of Isoflavones in Menopausal Health," *Menopause* 7 (2000): 215–29.

13. R. J. Miksicek, "Commonly Occurring Plant Flavonoids Have Estrogenic Activity," *Molecular Pharmacology* 44 (1993): 37–43.

14. L. U. Thompson et al., "Mammalian Lignan Production from Various Foods," *Nutrition and Cancer* 16 (1991): 43–52.

15. E. Ghisalberti, "Cardiovascular Activity of Naturally Occurring Lignans," *Phytomedicine* 4 (1997): 151–66.

16. K. Yamashita et al., "Sesamin and Alpha-Tocopherol Synergistically Suppress Lipid-Peroxide in Rats Fed a High Docosahexaenoic Acid Diet," *Biofactors* 11 (2000): 11–13.

17. M. Kojima et al., "Effect of KCA-098, a New Benzofuroquinoline Derivative, On Bone Mineral Metabolism," *Biological and Pharmaceutical Bulletin* 17 (1994): 504–8.

18. W. H. Utian, "Comparative Trial of P1496, a New Nonsteroidal Estrogen Analogue," *British Medical Journal* 1 (1973): 579–81.

19. T. Malini and G. Venithakumari, "Comparative Study of the Effects of Beta-Sitosterol, Estradiol, and Progesterone on Selected Biochemical

Parameters of the Uterus of Ovariectomized Rats," *Journal of Ethnopharmacology* 36 (1992): 51–55.

20. A. V. Rao and S. A. Janezic, "The Role of Dietary Phytosterols in Colon Carcinogenesis," *Nutrition and Cancer* 18 (1992): 43–52.

21. T. H. Burnham (ed.), *Gamma Oryzanol Monograph, The Review of Natural Products* (St. Louis, Mo.: Facts and Comparisons, September 1998).

22. N. Rong, L. M. Ausman, and R. J. Nicolosi, "Oryzanol Decreases Absorption and Aortic Fatty Streaks in Hamster," *Lipids* 32 (1997): 303–9.

23. J. B. Harborne and H. Baxter (eds.), *Phytochemical Dictionary* (Hampshire, England: Taylor and Francis Ltd., 1993).

24. P. Albertazzi, et al., "The Effect of Dietary Soy Supplementation on Hot Flushes," *Obstetrics and Gynecology* 91 (1998): 6–11.

25. D. C. Knight, P. L. Wall, and J. A. Eden, "A Review of Phytoestrogens and Their Effects in Relation to Menopausal Symptoms," *Australian Journal of Nutrition and Dietetics* 53 (1996): 5–11.

26. W. Zheng, Q. Dai, and L. J. Custer, "Urinary Excretion of Isoflavonoids and the Risk of Breast Cancer," *Cancer Epidemiology, Biomarkers, and Prevention* 8 (1999): 35–40.

27. A. R. Kennedy, "The Evidence for Soybean Products as Cancer Preventive Agents," *Journal of Nutrition* 125, Suppl. (1995): 733S–43S.

28. J. W. Anderson, B. M. Johnston, and M. E. Cook-Newell, "Meta-Analysis of the Effects of Soy Protein Intake on Serum Lipids," *New England Journal of Medicine* 333 (1995): 276–82.

29. T. H. Burnham (ed.), *Soy Monograph, The Review of Natural Products* (St. Louis, Mo.: Facts and Comparisons, September 1998).

30. D. C. Knight, J. A. Eden, and G. E. Kelly, "The Phytoestrogen Content of Infant Formulas," *Medical Journal of Australia* 164 (1996): 575.

31. A. Rzezinski et al., "Short-Term Effects of Phytoestrogen Rich Diet on Postmenopausal Women," *Journal of the North American Menopause Society* 4 (1997): 89–94.

32. D. D. Kitts et al., "Antioxidant Activity of the Flaxseed Lignan Secoisolariciresinal Diglycoside and Its Mammalian Lignan Metabolites

Enterodiol and Enterolactone," *Molecular and Cellular Biochemistry* 202 (2000): 91–100.

33. G. H. Arjmandi et al., "Whole Flax Seed Consumption Lowers Serum LDL Cholesterol and Lipoprotein Concentrations in Postmenopausal Women," *Nutrition Research* 18 (1998): 1203–14.

34. E. Ghisalberti, "Cardiovascular Activity of Naturally Occurring Lignans," *Phytomedicine* 4 (1997): 151–66.

35. M. Jenab et al., "Flaxseed and Lignans Increase Cecal Beta-Glucuronidase Activity in Rats," *Nutrition and Cancer* 33 (1999): 154–58.

36. L. U. Thompson et al., "Flaxseed and Its Lignan and Oil Components Reduce Mammary Tumor Growth at a Late Stage of Carcinogenesis," *Carcinogenesis* 17 (1996): 1373–76.

37. S. Cunnane, M. J. Hamadeh, and A. C. Liede, "Nutritional Attributes of Traditional Flaxseed in Healthy Young Adults," *American Journal of Clinical Nutrition* 61 (1995): 62–68.

38. W. J. Haggerty, "Flax: Ancient Herb and Modern Medicine," *HerbalGram* 45 (Winter 1999): 51–57.

39. S. M. Kingman, "The Influence of Legume Seeds on Human Plasma Lipid Concentrations," *Nutrition Research Reviews* 4 (1991): 97–123.

40. D. K. Salunkhe and S. S. Kadam (eds.), *CRC World Handbook of World Food Legumes: Nutritional Chemistry, Processing Technology, and Utilization* 2 (Boca Raton, Fla.: CRC Press, 1989).

41. J. Stavin, "Whole-Grain Consumption and Chronic Disease: Protective Mechanisms," *Nutrition and Cancer* 27 (1997): 14–21.

42. M. J. Davies et al., "Effects of Soy or Rye Supplementation of High-Fat Diets on Colon Tumor Development in Azoxymethane-Treated Rats," *Carcinogenesis* 20 (1999): 927–31.

43. K. R. Price and G. R. Fenwick, "Naturally Occurring Estrogens in Foods—A Review," *Food Additives and Contaminants* 2 (1985): 73–106.

44. J. Chury, "Ueber den Phytooestrogengehalt Einiger Pflanzen," *Experienta* 16 (1960): 194–59.

45. M. A. Zeligs, "Safer Estrogen with Phytonutrition," *Townsend Letter for Doctors and Patients* (April 1999): 83–88.

46. J. S. Gavaler et al., "Biologically Active Phytoestrogens Are Present in Bourbon," *Alcoholism: Clinical and Experimental Research* 11 (1987): 399–406.
47. D. H. Thiel et al., "The Phytoestrogens Present in De-Ethanolized Bourbon Are Biologically Active: A Preliminary Study in a Postmenopausal Woman," *Alcoholism: Clinical and Experimental Research* 15 (1991): 822–23.
48. H. Adlercreutz and W. Mazur, "Phytoestrogens and Western Diseases," *Annals of Medicine* 29 (1997): 95–120.

Chapter 4

1. J. Augustin et al., "Nutrient Content of Sprouted Wheat and Selected Legumes," *Cereal Foods World* 28 (1983): 358–61.
2. H. Chattopadhyay and S. Banerjee, "Effect of Germination on the Total Tocopherol Content of Pulses and Cereals," *Food Research* 17 (1952): 402–3.
3. P. L. Finney, "Effect of Germination on Cereal and Legume Nutrient Changes and Food or Feed Value: A Comprehensive Review," *Recent Advances in Phytochemistry* 17 (1983): 298.
4. D. K. Salunkhe and S. S. Kadam, *CRC Handbook of World Food Legumes: Nutritional Chemistry, Processing Technology, and Utilization* (Boca Raton, Fla.: CRC Press, 1989).
5. G. A. Rosenthal and P. Nkomo, "The Natural Abundance of L-Canavanine, an Active Anticancer Agent, in Alfalfa (Medicago sativa (L.)," *Pharmaceutical Biology* 38 (2000): 1–6.
6. T. Malini and G. Vanithakumari, "Comparative Study of the Effects of Beta-Sitosterol, Estradiol, and Progesterone on Selected Biochemical Parameters of the Uterus of Ovariectomized Rats," *Journal of Ethnopharmacology* 36 (1992): 51–55.
7. P. J. D. Bouie et al., "Beta-Sitosterol and Beta-Sitosterol Glucoside Stimulate Human Peripheral Blood Lymphocyte Proliferation: Implications for Their Use as an Immunomodulatory Vitamin Combination," *International Journal of Immunopharmacology* 18 (1996): 693–700.

Chapter 5

1. K. M. Lee et al., "Effects of *Humulus lupulus* Extract on the Central Nervous System in Mice," *Planta Medica* 59 (1993): A691.
2. British Herbal Medicine Association, *British Herbal Pharmacopoeia* (Cowling, U.K.: 1983).
3. T. Hudson, "Red Clover: A Review of its Use in the Menopausal Woman," *Townsend Letter for Doctors and Patients* (November 1999): 148–51.
4. P. Nestel et al., "Isoflavones in Red Clover May Reduce Coronary Vascular Disease Risk in Postmenopausal Women," *Journal of Clinical Endocrinology and Metabolism* 84 (1999): 895–98.
5. M. Blumenthal (ed.), *The Complete German Commission E Monographs* (Austin, Tex.: American Botanical Council, 1998).
6. F. C. Stoermer, R. Reistad, and J. Alexander, "Glycyrrhizic Acid in Liquorice—Evaluation of Health Hazard," *Food Chemical Toxicology* 31 (1993): 303–12.
7. E. M. Dueker et al., "Effects of Extracts from *Cimifuga racemosa* on Gonadotropin Release in Menopausal Women and Ovariectomized Rats," *Planta Medica* 57 (1991): 420–24.
8. J. Gruenwald, "Standardized Black Cohosh (Cimicifuga) Extract: Clinical Monograph," *Quarterly Review of Natural Medicine* (Summer 1998): 117–25.
9. H. W. Felter and J. U. Lloyd, *King's American Dispensatory*, vol. I (1898; reprint, Portland: Eclectic Medical Publications, Portland, 1983).
10. S. Foster, "Black Cohosh: *Cimicifuga racemosa*, a Literature Review," *HerbalGram* 45 (Winter 1999): 35–49.
11. G. Charalambous (ed.), *Spices, Herbs, and Edible Fungi* (New York: Elsevier, 1994).
12. M. Blumenthal (ed.), *The Complete German Commission E Monographs* (Austin, Tex.: American Botanical Council, 1998).
13. Committee on Food Protection, *Toxicants Occurring Naturally in Foods* (Washington, D.C.: National Academy of Sciences, 1973).
14. R. Punnonnen and A. Lukola, "Estrogen-like Effect of Ginseng," *The Lancet* 28 (1980): 1110.

15. V. D. Petkov et al., "Effects of Standardized Extracts GK402, from *Ginkgo biloba*, GI15 from *Panax ginseng*, and Their Combination, Gincosan, on the Brain Levels of Biogenic Monoamines and on the Serum Content of Prolactin, Growth Hormone, and ACTH," *Phytotherapy Research* 7 (1993): 139–45.

16. S. D. Elakovich and J. M. Hampton, "Analysis of Coumestrol, a Phytoestrogen in Alfalfa Tablets Sold for Human Consumption," *Journal of Agriculture and Food Chemistry* 32 (1984): 173–75.

17. M. Albert-Puleo, "Fennel and Anise as Estrogenic Agents," *Journal of Ethnopharmacology* 2 (1980): 377–84.

18. D. J. Brown, "Hawthorn—Phytotherapy Review and Commentary," *Townsend Letter for Doctors and Patients* (January 1996): 140–41.

19. E. Bombardelli and P. Morazzoni, "*Serenoa repens*," *Fitoterapia* 68 (1997): 99–113.

20. M. J. Elghamry and R. Haensel, "Activity and Isolated Phytoestrogen of Shrub Palmetto Fruits: A New Estrogenic Plant," *Experienta* 25 (1969): 828–29.

21. H. D. Reuter, K. J. Böhnert and U. Schmidt, "Treatment of Premenstrual Syndrome; Comparison of *Vitex agnus-castus* and Pyridoxine in a Controlled, Double Blind Study," *Quarterly Review of Natural Medicine* (Fall 1996): 187.

22. M. Blumenthal (ed.), *The Complete German Commission E Monographs* (Austin, Tex.: American Botanical Council, 1998).

23. J. D. Hirata et al., "Does Dong Quai Have Estrogenic Effects in Postmenopausal Women? A Double-Blind Placebo Controlled Trial," *Fertility and Sterility* 68 (1997): 981–86.

24. R. Chenoy et al., "Effect of Oral Gamma-Lenic Acid from Evening Primrose Oil on Menopausal Flushing," *British Medical Journal* 308 (1994): 501–3.

Chapter 6

1. S. Todorova et al., "Urinary Excretion of Glycosaminoglycans in Patients with Postmenopausal Osteoporosis," *Hormone Metabolism Research* 24 (1992): 585–87.

2. R. S. Weinstein and N. H. Bell, "Diminished Rates of Bone Formation in Normal Black Adults," *New England Journal of Medicine* 319 (1988): 1698–701.

3. L. Mosekilde and J. S. Thomsen, "Bone Structure and Function in Relation to Aging and the Menopause," in *Progress in the Management of the Menopause*, ed. B. G. Wren (New York: Parthenon, 1997), p. 134.

4. F. Branca, "Physical Activity, Diet, and Skeletal Health," *Public Health and Nutrition* 2 (1999): 391–96.

5. H. Malhus et al., "Excessive Dietary Intake of Vitamin A Is Associated with Reduced Bone Mineral Density and Increased Risk for Hip Fracture," *Annals of Internal Medicine* 129 (1998): 770–78.

6. G. Wyshak et al., "Nonalcoholic Carbonated Beverage Consumption and Bone Fractures among Women Former College Athletes," *Journal of Orthopedic Research* 7 (1989): 91–99.

7. R. E. Anderson et al., "Dieting Compromises Bone Density in Obese Women," *Metabolism* 8 (1997): 857–61.

8. M. Kishi et al., "Enhancing Effect of Dietary Vinegar on the Intestinal Absoprtion of Calcium in Ovariectomized Rats," *Bioscience, Biotechnology, and Biochemistry* 63 (1999): 905–10.

9. M. B. Roberfroid, "Prebiotics and Synbiotics: Concepts and Nutritional Properties," *British Journal of Nutrition* 80, Suppl. (1998): S197–S202.

10. P. D. O'Loughlin and H. A. Morris, "Calcium Homeostasis and Osteoporosis," *Clinical Biochemistry Reviews* 19 (1998): 3–17.

11. L. Cobiac, *Lactose: A Review of Intakes and of Importance to Health of Australians and New Zealanders* (Adelaide: CSIRO Division of Human Nutrition, 1994).

12. D. Pearson and L. McTaggart, "Osteoporosis: A Load of Old Bones," *Control Your Health* 6 (1996): 1–3.

13. H. Melhus et al., "Smoking, Antioxidant Vitamins, and the Risk of Hip Fracture," *Journal of Bone and Mineral Research* 14 (1999): 129–35.

14. A. F. Jorm et al., "Smoking and Mental Health: Results from a Community Survey," *Medical Journal of Australia* 170 (1999): 74–77.

15. A. Sebastian et al., "Improved Mineral Balance and Skeletal Metabolism in Postmenopausal Women Treated With Potassium Bicarbonate," *New England Journal of Medicine* 330 (1994): 1776–81, (three reports).

16. *Journal of Nutrition* 128 (1998): 1048–57.

17. J. F. Chiu et al., "Long-Term Vegetarian Diet and Bone Mineral Density in Postmenopausal Taiwanese Women," *Calcified Tissue International* 60 (1997): 245–49.

18. M. A. Schürch et al., "Protein Supplements Increase Serum Insulin-Like Growth Factor-I Levels and Attenuate Proximal Femur Bone Loss in Patients with Recent Hip Fracture," *Archives of Internal Medicine* 128 (1998): 801–9.

19. F. T. Cappuccio et al., "A Prospective Study of Blood Pressure and Bone Mineral Loss in Elderly White Women: The Study of Osteoporotic Fractures," *Circulation* 98, Suppl. (1998): S1657.

20. U. N. Nguyen et al., "Aspartame Ingestion Increases Urinary Calcium but Not Oxalate Excretion in Healthy Subjects," *Journal of Clinical Endocrinology and Metabolism* 83 (1998): 165–68.

21. M. S. Calva and Y. K. Park, "Changing Phosphorus Content of the U.S. Diet: Potential for Adverse Effects on Bone," *Journal of Nutrition* 126 (1996): 1168S–1180S.

22. A. Tavani et al., "Coffee Intake and Risk of Hip Fracture in Women in Northern Italy," *Preventive Medicine* 24 (1995): 396–400.

23. A. Tavani et al., "Calcium, Dairy Products, and the Risk of Hip Fracture in Women in Northern Italy," *Epidemiology* 6 (1995): 554–57.

24. A. W. Burgstahler and J. Colquhoun, "Neurotoxicity of Fluoride," *Fluoride* 29 (1996): 57–58.

25. J. R. Lee, "Fluoridation and Hip Fracture," *Fluoride* 26 (1993): 274–77.

26. R. W. Porter et al., "Prediction of Hip Fracture in Elderly Women: A Prospective Study," *British Medical Journal* 301 (1990): 638–41.

27. P. J. Kelly et al., "Dietary Calcium, Sex Hormones, and Bone Mineral Density in Men," *British Medical Journal* 300 (1990): 1361–62.

28. J. R. Center et al., "Mortality after All Major Types of Osteoporotic Fracture in Men and Women: An Observational Study," *The Lancet* 353 (1999): 878–82.

29. A. Trichopoulou et al., "Energy Intake and Monounsaturated Fat in Relation to Bone Mineral Density among Women and Men in Greece," *Preventive Medicine* 26 (1997): 395–400.

30. M. R. Law et al., "Preventing Osteoporosis," *British Medical Journal* 383 (1991): 922.
31. D. T. Felson et al., "The Effect of Postmenopausal Estrogen Therapy on Bone Density in Elderly Women," *New England Journal of Medicine* 329 (1993): 1141–46.
32. B. L. Riggs and L. J. Melton, "The Prevention and Treatment of Osteoporosis," *New England Journal of Medicine* 327 (1992): 620–27.
33. N. F. Col, "Individualizing Therapy to Prevent Long-Term Consequences of Estrogen Deficiency in Postmenopausal Women," *Archives of Internal Medicine* 159 (1999): 1458–66.
34. E. Seeman, "Osteoporosis: Treatment Options," in *Progress in the Management of the Menopause*, ed. B. G. Wren (New York: Parthenon, 1997).
35. H. Leonetti et al., "Transdermal Progesterone Cream for Vasomotor Symptoms and Postmenopausal Bone Loss," *Obstetrics and Gynecology* 94 (1999): 225–28.
36. C. Gennari et al., "Effect of Chronic Treatment with Ipriflavone in Postmenopausal Women with Low Bone Mass," *Calcified Tissue International* 61, Suppl. (1997): S19–S22.
37. B. Kass-Annese, "Alternative Therapies for Menopause," *Clinical Obstetrics and Gynecology* 43 (2000): 162–83.
38. S. J. Wimalawansa, "Combined Therapy with Estrogen and Etidronate Has an Additive Effect on Bone Mineral Density in the Hip and Vertebrae: Four-Year Randomized Study," *American Journal of Medicine* 99 (1995): 36–42.
39. S. R. Davis et al., "Testosterone Enhances Estradiol's Effects on Postmenopausal Bone Density and Sexuality," *Maturitas* 21 (1995): 226–36.

Chapter 7

1. A. Hartmann et al., "Vitamin E Prevents Exercise-Induced DNA Damage," *Mutation Research* 346 (1995): 195–202.
2. G. A. Bachmann and J. Grill, "Exercise in the Postmenopausal Woman," *Geriatrics* 42 (1987): 75–85.
3. R. Marcus et al., "Osteoporosis and Exercise in Women," *Medicine and Science in Sports and Exercise* 24, Suppl. (1992): S301–7.

4. M. Notelovitz, "An Opposing View," *Journal of Family Practice* 29 (1989): 410–15.

5. K. A. Grove and B. R. Londeree, "Bone Density in Postmenopausal Women: High Impact Versus Low Impact Exercise," *Medicine and Science in Sports and Exercise* 24 (1992): 1190–94.

6. S. H. Guelder et al., "Long-Term Exercise Patterns and Immune Function in Healthy Older Women: A Report of Preliminary Findings," *Mechanisms of Ageing and Development* 93 (1997): 215–22.

7. D. R. Seals et al., "Effects of Regular Aerobic Exercise on Elevated Blood Pressure in Postmenopausal Women," *American Journal of Cardiology* 80 (1997): 49–55.

8. I. M. Lee et al., "Exercise Intensity and Longevity in Men," *Journal of the American Medical Association* 273 (1995): 1179–84.

9. O. G. Cameron and C. J. Hudson, "Influence of Exercise on Anxiety Level in Patients with Anxiety Disorders," *Psychosomatics* 27 (1986): 720–21.

10. W. Aldoori et al., "A Prospective Study of Physical Activity and the Risk of Symptomatic Diverticular Disease in Men," *American Journal of Epidemiology* 139, Suppl. (1994): S35.

11. M. F. Leitzmann et al., "Recreational Physical Activity and the Risk of Cholecystectomy in Women," *New England Journal of Medicine* 341 (1999): 77–84.

12. M. S. Passo et al., "Exercise Training Reduces Intraocular Pressure among Subjects Suspected of Having Glaucoma," *Archives of Ophthalmology* 109 (1991): 1096–98.

13. M. Pantaleoni et al., "Changes in the Blood Levels of Adrenal Hormones after Prolonged Physical Activity," *Minerva Endrocinology* 16 (2000): 17–20.

14. W. J. Evans, "Effects of Aging and Exercise on Nutrition Needs of the Elderly," *Nutrition Reviews* 54 (1996): S35–39.

15. M. A. Fiatarone et al., "High-Intensity Strength Training in Nonagenarians: Effects on Skeletal Muscle," *Journal of the American Medical Association* 263 (1990): 3029–34.

16. A. MacIntosh, "Exercise and Osteoporosis," *Townsend Letter for Doctors & Patients* (November 1995): 46.

17. B. A. Michel et al., "Effect of Changes in Weight-Bearing Exercise on Lumbar Bone Mass after Age Fifty," *Annals of Medicine* 23 (1991): 397–401.

18. J. M. Bell and E. J. Bassey, "Postexercise Heart Rates and Pulse Palpation as a Means of Determining Exercising Intensity in an Aerobic Dance Class," *British Journal of Sports and Medicine* 30 (1996): 48–52.

19. R. T. Cotton (ed.), *Exercise for Older Adults*, San Diego, Calif.:, American Council on Exercise, 1998.

20. K. Narita et al., "Development and Evaluation of a New Target Heart Rate Formula for the Adequate Exercise Training Level in Healthy Subjects," *Journal of Cardiology* 33 (1999): 265–72.

Chapter 8

1. L. Strause et al., "Spinal Bone Loss with Postmenopausal Women Supplemented with Calcium and Trace Minerals," *Journal of Nutrition* 124 (1994): 1060–64.

2. D. Pearson and L. McTaggart, "Osteoporosis: A Load of Old Bones," *Control Your Health* 6 (1992): 2–3.

3. A. Prentice, "Is Nutrition Important in Osteoporosis?" *Proceedings of the Nutrition Society* 56 (1997): 357–67.

4. D. Feskanich et al., "Vitamin K Intake and Hip Fractures in Women: A Prospective Study," *American Journal of Clinical Nutrition* 69 (1999): 74–79.

5. M. C. Wang et al., "Associations of Vitamin C, Calcium, and Protein with Bone Mass in Postmenopausal Mexican American Women," *Osteoporosis International* 7 (1996): 533–38.

6. H. Melhus et al., "Smoking, Antioxidant Vitamins, and the Risk of Hip Fracture," *Journal of Bone and Mineral Research* 14 (1999): 129–35.

7. S. A. New et al., "Dietary Influences on Bone Mass and Bone Metabolism: Further Evidence of a Positive Link between Fruit and Vegetable Consumption and Bone Health?" *American Journal of Clinical Nutrition* 71 (2000): 142–51.

8. N. J. Lemann Jr. et al., "Potassium Causes Calcium Retention in Healthy Adults," *Journal of Nutrition* 123 (1993): 1623–26.

9. S. M. Potter et al., "Soy Protein and Isoflavones: Their Effects on Blood Lipids and Bone Density in Postmenopausal Women," *American Journal of Clinical Nutrition* 68, Suppl. (1998): 1357S–79S.

10. J. McLaren-Howard, E. C. G. Grant, and S. Davies, "Hormone Replacement Therapy and Osteoporosis: Bone Enzymes and Nutrient Imbalances," *Journal of Nutrition and Environmental Medicine* 8 (1998): 126–38.

11. J. Eaton-Evans, "Osteoporosis and the Role of Diet," *British Journal of Biomedical Science* 54 (1994): 358–70.

12. M. A. Schurch et al., "Protein Supplements Increase Serum Insulin-Like Growth Factor-I Levels and Attenuate Proximal Femur Bone Loss in Patients with a Recent Hip Fracture: A Randomized Double Blind Placebo Controlled Trial," *Annals of Internal Medicine* 128 (1998): 801–9.

13. A. Prentice, "Is Nutrition Important in Osteoporosis?" *Proceedings of the Nutrition Society* 56 (1997): 357–67.

14. J. McLaren, E. C. G. Grant, and S. Davies, "Hormone Replacement Therapy and Osteoporosis: Bone Enzymes and Nutrient Imbalances," *Journal of Nutritional and Environmental Medicine* 8 (1998): 129–38.

15. M. C. Kruger et al., "Calcium, Gamma-Linolenic Acid and Eicosapentaenoic Acid Supplementation in Senile Osteopororis," *Aging* 10 (1998): 385–94.

16. G. Van Papendorp. B. Coetzer, and M. Kruger, "Biochemical Profile of Osteoporotic Patients on Essential Fatty Acid Supplementation," *Nutrition Research* 15 (1995): 325–34.

17. H. Xu, B. A. Watkins, and M. F. Seifert, "Vitamin E Stimulates Trabecular Bone Formation and Alters Epiphyseal Cartilage Morphometry," *Calcified Tissue International* 57 (1995): 293–300.

18. G. Stendig-Lindberg et al., "Trabecular Bone Density in a Two Year Controlled Trial of Peroral Magnesium in Osteoporosis," *Magnesium Research* 6 (1993): 155–63.

19. J. E. Sojka and C. M. Weaver, "Magnesium Supplementation and Osteoporosis," *Nutrition Reviews* 53 (1995): 71–74.

20. E. Grant, *Sexual Chemistry* (London: Cedar, 1994).
21. M. S. Seelig, "Increased Need for Magnesium with the Use of Combined Estrogen and Calcium for Osteoporosis Treatment," *Magnesium Research* 3 (1990): 197–215.
22. G. E. Abraham and H. Grewal, "A Total Dietary Program Emphasizing Magnesium Instead of Calcium: Effect on the Mineral Density of Calcaneous Bone in Postmenopausal Women on Hormonal Therapy," *Journal of Reproductive Medicine* 35 (1990): 503–07.
23. G. E. Abraham, "The Importance of Magnesium in the Management of Primary Postmenopausal Osteoporosis," *Journal of Nutritional Medicine* 2 (1991): 165–78.
24. C. D. Hunt, J. L. Herbel, and F. H. Nielsen, "Metabolic Responses of Postmenopausal Women to Supplemental Dietary Boron and Aluminum During Usual and Low Magnesium Intake: Boron, Calcium, and Magnesium Absorption and Retention and Blood Mineral Concentrations," *American Journal of Clinical Nutrition* 65 (1997): 803–13.
25. A. R. Gaby and J. V. Wright, "Nutrients and Osteoporosis," *Journal of Nutritional Medicine* 1 (1990): 63–72.
26. M. R. Naghii and S. Samman, "The Role of Boron in Nutrition and Metabolism," *Progress in Food and Nutrition Science* 17 (1993): 331–49.
27. R. L. Travers, G. C. Rennie, and R. E. Newnham, "Boron and Arthritis: The Result of a Double-Blind Pilot Study," *Journal of Nutritional Medicine* 1 (1990): 127–32.
28. F. H. Nielsen, "Studies on the Relationship Between Boron and Magnesium which Possibly Affects the Formation and Maintenance of Bones," *Magnesium and Trace Elements* 9 (1990): 61–69.
29. F. H. Nielsen, "Boron in Human and Animal Nutrition," *Plant and Soil* 193 (1997): 199–208.
30. E. Grant, *Sexual Chemistry* (London: Cedar, 1994).
31. J. Brandae-Neto et al., "The Essential Role of Zinc in Growth," *Nutrition Research* 14 (1995): 335–38.
32. E. Grant, *Sexual Chemistry* (London: Cedar, 1994).

33. N. Loveridge and B. S. Noble, "Control of Longitudinal Growth: The Role of Nutrition," *European Journal of Clinical Nutrition* 48 (1994): 74–84.

34. J. Jonas et al., "Impaired Mechanical Strength of Bone in Experimental Copper Deficiency," *Annals of Nutrition and Metabolism* 37 (1993): 245–52.

35. C. D. Seaborn and F. H. Nielsen, "Silicon: A Nutritional Beneficence for Bones, Brains, and Blood Vessels?" *Nutrition Today* (July/August 1993): 13–18.

36. J. H. Beattie and A. Avenell, "Trace Element Nutrition and Bone Metabolism," *Nutrition Research Reviews* 5 (1992): 167–88.

37. A. R. Gaby and J. V. Wright, "Nutrients and Osteoporosis," *Journal of Nutritional Medicine* 1 (1990): 63–72.

38. J. McLaren-Howard, E. C. G. Grant, and S. Davies, "Hormone Replacement Therapy and Osteoporosis: Bone Enzymes and Nutrient Imbalances," *Journal of Nutritional and Environmental Medicine* 8 (1998): 129–38.

39. E. Grant, *Sexual Chemistry* (London: Cedar, 1994).

40. G. S. Kim et al., "Effects of Vitamin B_{12} on Cell Proliferation and Cellular Alkaline Phosphatase Activity in Human Bone Marrow Stromal Osteoprogenitor Cells and UMR106 Osteoblastic Cells," *Metabolism: Clinical and Experimental* 45 (1996): 1443–46.

41. M. Chapuy, "Vitamin D and Calcium to Prevent Hip Fractures in Elderly Women, *New England Journal of Medicine* 327 (1992): 1636–42.

42. K. T. Khaw, M. J. Sneyd, and J. Compstone, "Bone Density, Parathyroid Hormone, and 25-Hydroxyvitamin D Concentrations in Middle Aged Women," *British Medical Journal* 305 (1992): 273–77.

43. J. A. Kanis, "Calcium Nutrition and Its Implications for Osteoporosis, Part I," *European Journal of Clinical Nutrition* 48 (1994): 757–67.

44. M. Chapuy and P. J. Meunier, "Prevention of Secondary Hyperparathy-roidism and Hip Fracture in Elderly Women with Calcium and Vitamin D_3 Supplements," *Osteoporosis International* 6 (1996): 60–63.

45. J. E. Sojka and C. M. Weaver, "Magnesium Supplementation and Osteoporosis," *Nutrition Reviews* 53 (1995): 72–80.

46. J. W. Nieves et al., "Calcium Potentiates the Effect of Estrogen and Calcitonin on Bone Mass: Review and Analysis," *American Journal of Clinical Nutrition* 67 (1998): 18–24.

47. S. B. Eaton, M. Shostak, and M. Konner, *The Paleolithic Prescription: A Program of Diet and Exercise and a Design for Living* (New York: Harper and Row, 1988).

48. M. Annefeld et al., "The Influence of Ossein-Hydroxyapatite Compound on the Healing of a Bone Defect," *Current Medical Research and Opinion* 10 (1986): 241–50.

49. L. Patrick, "Comparative Absorption of Calcium Sources and Calcium Citrate Malate for the Prevention of Osteoporosis," *Alternative Medicine Review* 4 (1999): 74–85.

50. J. F. Hu et al., "Dietary Intakes and Urinary Excretion of Calcium and Acids: A Cross-Sectional Study of Women in China," *American Journal of Clinical Nutrition* 58 (1993): 398–406.

51. P. D. Saltman and L. G. Strause, "The Role of Trace Minerals in Osteoporosis," *Journal of the American College of Nutrition* 12 (1993): 384–89.

52. J. McLaren, E. C. G. Grant, and S. Davies, "Hormone Replacement Therapy and Osteoporosis: Bone Enzymes and Nutrient Imbalances," *Journal of Nutritional and Environmental Medicine* 8 (1998): 129–38.

Chapter 9

1. J. T. Salonen et al., "Donation of Blood is Associated with Reduced Risk of Myocardial Infarction. The Kuopio Ischaemic Heart Disease Risk Factor Study," *American Journal of Epidemiology* 148 (1998): 445–51.

2. F. B. Hu et al., "Frequent Nut Consumption and Risk of Coronary Heart Disease in Women: Prospective Cohort Study," *British Medical Journal* 317 (1998): 1341–45.

3. P. Wehrwein, "More Evidence That Tea Is Good for the Heart," *The Lancet* 353 (1999): 384.

4. R. B. Singh et al., "Randomized Double Blind Placebo Controlled Trial of Coenzyme Q10 in Patients with Acute Myocardial Infarction," *Cardiovascular Drugs and Therapy* 12 (1998): 347–53.

5. T. H. Burnham (ed.), *Lecithin Monograph, Review of Natural Products* (St. Louis, Mo.: Facts and Comparisons, September 1998).

6. Homocysteine Lowering Trialists' Collaboration, "Lowering Blood Homocysteine with Folic Acid Based Supplements: Meta-Analysis of Randomized Trials," *British Medical Journal* 316 (1998): 894–98.

7. O. Nygard et al., "Coffee Consumption and Plasma Total Homocysteine: The Hordaland Homocysteine Study," *American Journal of Clinical Nutrition* 65 (1997): 136–43.

8. G. P. Oakley, "Eat Right and Take a Multivitamin," *New England Journal of Medicine* 338 (1998): 775.

9. F. Kiao, A. R. Folsom, and F. L. Brancati, "Is Low Magnesium Concentration a Risk Factor for Coronary Heart Disease? The Atherosclerosis Risk in Communities Study," *American Heart Journal* 136 (1998): 480–90.

10. D. J. Brown, "Hawthorn—Phytotherapy Review and Commentary," *Townsend Letter for Doctors and Patients* (January 1996): 140–41.

11. S. Dwivedi and R. Jauhari, "Beneficial Effects of *Terminalia arjuna* in Coronary Artery Disease," *Indian Heart Journal* 49 (1997): 507–10.

12. J. Shen et al., "Effects of EGb761 on Nitric Oxide and Oxygen Free Radicals, Myocardial Damage, and Arrhythmia in Ischemia-Reperfusion Injury in Vivo," *Biochimica et Biophysica Acta* 1406 (1998): 228–36.

13. S. B. Kritchevsky et al., "Provitamin A Carotenoid Intake and Carotid Artery Plaque: The Atherosclerosis Risk in Communities Study," *American Journal of Clinical Nutrition* 68 (1998): 726–33.

14. T. R. Watkins and M. L. Bierenbaum, "Grape Juice Attenuates Cardiovascular Risk Factors in the Hyperlipemic Subject," *Pharmaceutical Biology* 36, Suppl. (1998): 75–80.

15. C. A. Chan, "Vitamin E and Atherosclerosis," *Journal of Nutrition* 128 (1998): 1593–96.

16. P. J. Davey et al., "Cost-Effectiveness of Vitamin E Therapy in the Treatment of Patients with Angiographically Proven Coronary Narrowing (CHAOS trial)," *American Journal of Cardiology* 82 (1998): 414–17.

17. L. A. Simons, M. Von Konigsmark, and S. Balasubrahmaniam, "What Dose of Vitamin E Is Required to Reduce Susceptibility of LDL to

Oxidation?" *Australian and New Zealand Medical Journal* 26 (1996): 496–503.

18. J. C. Peterson, "Vitamins and Progression of Atherosclerosis in Hyper-homocysteinemia," *The Lancet* 351 (1998): 263.

19. J. T. Salonen et al., "Lipoprotein Oxidation and Progression of Carotid Atherosclerosis," *Circulation* 95 (1997): 840–45.

20. S. R. Wenneberg et al., "Anger Expression Correlates with Platelet Aggregation," *Behavioral Medicine* 22 (1997): 174–77.

21. F. M. Luskin et al., "A Review of Mind-Body Therapies in the Treatment of Cardiovascular Disease. Part I: Implications for the Elderly," *Alternative Therapies in Health and Medicine* 4 (1998): 46–61.

22. J. W. Anderson, B. M. Johnstone, and M. E. Cook-Newell, "Meta-Analysis of the Effects of Soy Protein Intake on Serum Lipids," *New England Journal of Medicine* 333 (1995): 276–82.

23. M. J. Tikkanen et al., "Effect of Soybean Phytoestrogens Intake on Low Density Lipoprotein Oxidation Resistance," *Proceedings of the National Academy of Sciences USA* 95 (1998): 3106–10.

24. U. Arens, "Reasons Not to Be Cheerful" *BNF Bulletin* 21 (1996): 93–94.

25. R. H. Schneider et al., "Lower Lipid Peroxide Levels in Practitioners of the Transcendental Mediation Program," *Psychosomatic Medicine* 60 (1998): 38–41.

26. J. S. Naruka, R. Mathur, and A. Mathur, "Effect of Pranayama Practices on Fasting Blood Glucose and Serum Cholesterol," *Indian Journal of Medical Sciences* 40 (1986): 149–52.

27. L. J. Appel et al., "A Clinical Trial of the Effects of Dietary Patterns on Blood Pressure," *New England Journal of Medicine* 336 (1997): 1117–24.

28. Y. Kawano et al., "Effects of Magnesium Supplementation in Hypertensive Patients," *Hypertension* 32 (1998): 250–65.

29. D. R. Seals et al., "Effect of Regular Aerobic Activity on Elevated Blood Pressure in Postmenopausal Women," *American Journal of Cardiology* 80 (1997): 49–55.

30. S. R. Wenneberg et al., "A Controlled Study of the Effects of the Transcendental Meditation Program on Cardiovascular Reactivity and

Ambulatory Blood Pressure," *International Journal of Neuroscience* 89 (1997): 15–28.

31. S. A. Everson et al., "Hopelessness and 4-Year Progression of Carotid Atherosclerosis," *Arteriosclerosis, Thrombosis, and Vascular Biology* 17 (1997): 1490–95.

32. K. J. Joshipura et al., "Fruit and Vegetable Intake in Relation to Risk of Ischemic Stroke," *Journal of the American Medical Association* 282 (1999): 1233–39.

33. H. B. Van der Worp et al., "Protective Effect of Vitamin E in a Rat Model of Focal Cerebral Ischemia," *Stroke* 29 (1998): 1002–06.

34. A. Bordia et al., "Effect of Ginger and Fenugreek on Blood Lipids, Blood Sugar, and Platelet Aggregation in Patients with Coronary Artery Disease," *Prostaglandins, Leukotrienes, and Essential Fatty Acids* 56 (1997): 379–84.

35. A. K. Kaung et al., "Long-Term Observation on Qijong in Prevention of Stroke—Follow-Up of 244 Hypertensive Patients for 18–22 Years," *Journal of Traditional Chinese Medicine* 6 (1986): 235–38.

36. G. A. Lammie et al., "Stress-Related Primary Intracerebral Hemorrhage: Autopsy Clues to Underlying Mechanism," *Stroke* 31 (2000): 1426–28.

37. W. H. Aldoori et al., "Use of Acetaminophen and Nonsteroidal Anti-Inflammatory Drugs," *Archives of Family Medicine* 7 (1998): 255–60.

38. P. L. Le Bars et al., "A Placebo Controlled Double Blind Randomized Trial of an Extract for Dementia: North American EGb Study Group," *Journal of the American Medical Association* 278 (1997): 1327–32.

39. K. Winther et al., "Effect of Ginkgo biloba Extract on Cognitive Function and Blood Pressure in Elderly Subjects," *Current Therapeutic Research* 59 (1998): 881–88.

40. M. C. Morris et al., "Vitamin E and Vitamin C Supplement Use and Risk of Incident Alzheimer Disease," *Alzheimer Disease and Associated Disorders* 12 (1998): 121–26.

41. K. Van Dyke, "The Possible Role of Peroxynitrite in Alzheimer's Disease: A Simple Hypothesis That Could Be Tested More Thoroughly," *Medical Hypotheses* 48 (1997): 375–80.

42. M. Sano et al., "A Controlled Trial of Selegiline, Alpha-Tocopherol, or Both as a Treatment for Alzheimer's Disease," *The New England Journal of Medicine* 336 (1997): 1216–22.

43. A. L. Stoll et al., "Omega-3 Fatty Acids in Bipolar Disorder: A Preliminary Double Blind Placebo Controlled Trial," *Archives of General Psychiatry* 56 (1999): 407–12.

44. P. Kidd, "Phosphatidylserine: Membrane Nutrient for Memory—a Clinical and Mechanistic Assessment," *Alternative Medicine Reviews* 1 (1996): 70–84.

45. P. M. Doraiswamy and D. C. Steffens, "Combination Therapy for Early Alzheimer's Disease: What Are We Waiting For?" *Journal of the American Geriatric Society* 46 (1998): 1322–24.

46. R. B. McDonald, "Influence of Dietary Sucrose on Biological Aging," *American Journal of Clinical Nutrition* 62 (1995): 284–93.

47. A. B. Caragay, "Cancer-Preventive Foods and Ingredients," *Food Technology* 46 (1992): 65–68.

48. J. L. Freudenheim et al., "Premenopausal Breast Cancer Risk and Intake of Vegetables, Fruits, and Related Nutrients," *Journal of the National Cancer Institute* 88 (1996): 340–48.

49. B. L. Pool-Zobel et al., "Consumption of Vegetables Reduces Genetic Damage in Humans: First Results of a Human Intervention Trial with Carotenoid-Rich Foods," *Carcinogenesis* 18 (1997): 1847–50.

50. S. Choi and J. Mayer, "Vitamin B_{12} Deficiency: A New Risk Factor for Breast Cancer?" *Nutrition Reviews* 57 (1999): 250–53.

51. S. L. Romney et al., "Nutrient Antioxidants in the Pathogenesis and Prevention of Cervical Dysplasia and Cancer," *Journal of Cellular Biochemistry* 23 (1995): 96–103.

52. J. H. Cummings and S. A. Bingham, "Diet and the Prevention of Cancer," *British Medical Journal* 317 (1998): 1636–40.

53. K. N. Prasad et al., "High Doses of Multiple Antioxidant Vitamins: Essential Ingredients in Improving the Efficacy of Standard Cancer Therapy," *Journal of the American College of Nutrition* 18 (1999): 13–25.

54. D. W. Lamson and M. S. Brignall, "Antioxidants in Cancer Therapy: Their Actions and Interactions with Oncological Therapies," *Alternative Medicine Reviews* 4 (1999): 304–29.

55. C. A. Gogos et al., "Dietary Omega-3 Polyunsaturated Fatty Acids Plus Vitamin E Restore Immunodeficiency and Prolong Survival for Severely Ill Patients with Generalized Malignancy," *Cancer* 82 (1998): 395–402.
56. Y. J. Hu, "The Protective Role of Selenium on the Toxicity of Cisplatin-Contained Chemotherapy Regimen in Cancer Patients," *Biological Trace Element Research* 56 (1997): 331–41.

Chapter 10

1. S. Telles and K. V. Naveen, "Yoga for Rehabilitation: An Overview," *Indian Journal of Medical Science* 51 (1997): 123–27.
2. K. M. Dillon, B. Minchoff, and K. H. Baker, "Positive Emotional States and Enhancement of the Immune System," *International Journal of Psychiatric Medicine* 15 (1985): 13–17.
3. C. R. MacLean et al., "Effects of the Transcendental Meditation Program on Adaptive Mechanisms: Changes in Hormone Levels and Responses to Stress after Four Months of Practice," *Psychoneurendocrinology* 22 (1997): 277–95.
4. T. Maruta et al., "Optimists Versus Pessimists: Survival Rate Among Medical Patients," *Mayo Clinic Proceedings* 75 (2000): 140–43.
5. Thich Nhat Hanh, *The Miracle of Mindfulness* (Boston: Beacon Press, 1995).
6. J. A. Astin, "Stress Reduction through Mindfulness Meditation: Effects on Psychological Symptomatology, Sense of Control, and Spiritual Experiences," *Psychotherapy and Psychosomatics* 66 (1997): 97–106.
7. S. O'Laoire, "An Experimental Study of the Effects of Distant, Intercessory Prayer on Self-Esteem, Anxiety, and Depression," *Alternative Therapies in Health and Medicine* 3 (1997): 38–53.
8. H. G. Koenig et al., "The Relationship Between Religious Activities and Blood Pressure in Older Adults," *International Journal of Psychiatry in Medicine* 28 (1998): 189–213.
9. G. Searle, *Stillness Be My Friend* (Homebush, NSW, Australia: St. Paul's, 1998).
10. R. J. Williams, *You are Extraordinary* (New York: Pyramid Books, 1976, p. 257.

11. Dalai Lama, *The World of Tibetan Buddhism* (Boston: Wisdom Publications, 1995).

12. R. H. Schneider et al., "Lower Lipid Peroxide Levels in Practitioners of the Transcendental Meditation Program," *Psychosomatic Medicine* 60 (1998): 38–41.

13. J. L. Glaser et al., "Elevated Serum Dehydroepiandrosterone Sulfate Levels in Practitioners of the Transcendental Meditation (TM) and TM-Sidhi Programs," *Journal of Behavioral Medicine* 15 (1992): 327–41.

14. D. Orme-Johnson, "Medical Care Utilization and the Transcendental Meditation Program," *Psychosomatic Medicine* 49 (1987): 493-507.

Chapter 11

1. A. Køster and K. Garde, "Sexual Desire and Menopausal Development," *Maturitas* 161 (1993): 49–60.

2. G. S. Bachmann and S. R. Leiblum, "Sexuality in Sexagenarian Women," *Maturitas* 13 (1991): 43–50.

3. S. A. Kingsberg, "Postmenopausal Sexual Functioning: A Case Study," *International Journal of Fertility and Women's Medicine* 43 (1998): 122–28.

4. A. Collins and B. M. Landgren, "Psychosocial Factors Associated with the Use of Hormonal Replacement Therapy in a Longitudinal Follow-up of Swedish Women," *Maturitas* 28 (1997): 1–9.

5. B. Seaman and G. Seaman, *Women and the Crisis in Sex Hormones* (Sussex, England: Harvester Press, 1978).

6. E. Laan and R. H. van Lunsen, "Hormones and Sexuality in Postmenopausal Women: A Psychophysiological Study," *Journal Psychosomatic Obstetrics and Gynaecology* 18 (1997): 126–33.

7. R. C. Rosen et al., "Prevalence of Sexual Dysfunction in Women: Results of a Survey Study of 320 Women in an Outpatient Gynecological Clinic," *Journal Sex and Marital Therapy* 19 (1993): 171–88.

8. G. Greer, *The Change* (London: Hamish Hamilton, 1991).

9. R. G. Kennedy, T. Davies, and F. Al-Azzawi, "Sexual Interest in Postmenopausal Women Is Related to 5-alpha-reductase Activity," *Human Reproduction* 12 (1997): 209–13.

10. A. Zeleniuch-Jacquotte, P. F. Bruning, and J. M. Bonfrer, "Relation of Serum Levels of Testosterone and Dehydroepiandronsterone Sulfate to Risk of Breast Cancer in Postmenopausal Women," *American Journal of Epidemiology* 145 (1997): 1030–38.
11. A. Grazziottin, "Hormones and Libido," in *Progress in the Management of the Menopause*, ed. B. G. Wren (New York: Parthenon, 1996).
12. R. G. Berg et al., "Hormal Replacement Therapy and Sexuality in a Population of Swedish Postmenopausal Women," *Acta Obstetrica et Gynecologica Scandinavica* 72 (1993): 282–97.
13. S. Leiblum et al., "Vaginal Atrophy in the Postmenopausal Woman. The Importance of Sexual Activity and Hormones," *Journal of the American Medical Association* 249 (2000): 2195–98.
14. R. Raz and W. E. Stamm, "A Controlled Trial of Intravaginal Estriol in Postmenopausal Women with Recurrent Urinary Tract Infections," *New England Journal of Medicine* 329 (1993): 753–56.
15. M. J. Pearce and K. Hawton, "Psychological and Sexual Aspects of the Menopause and HRT," *Baillieres Clinical Obstetrics and Gynaecology* 10 (1996): 385–99.

Appendix III

1. C. M. Dollbaum, "Lab Analyses of Salivary DHEA and Progesterone Following Ingestion of Yam-Containing Products," *Townsend Letter for Doctors & Patients* (October 1996): 104.
2. M. Araghiniknam et al., "Antioxidant Activity of Dioscorea and Dehydroepiandrosterone (DHEA) in Older Humans," *Life Sciences* 59 (1996): 147–57.
3. G. Mirkin, "Estrogen in Yams," *Journal of the American Medical Association* 265 (1991); 912.
4. D. G. Coursey, *Yams* (London: Longmans, 1967).
5. G. Blunden and R. Hardman, "Quantitative Estimation of Diosgenin in Dioscorea Tubers by Densitometric Thin-Layer Chromatography," *Journal of Pharmaceutical Sciences* 56 (1967): 948–50.

6. G. Blunden and C. T. Rhodes, "Stability of Diosgenin," *Journal of Pharmaceutical Sciences* 57 (1968): 602–04.

7. M. S. Ross and K. R. Brain, *An Introduction to Phytopharmacy* (London: Pitman Medical, 1977).

8. A. Rao, A. R. Rao, and R. K. Kale, "Diosgenin—A Growth Stimulator of Mammary Gland of Ovariectomized Mouse," *Indian Journal of Experimental Biology* 30 (1992): 367–70.

9. P. Komesaroff, "Results of Study of Effects of Wild Yam Extract in Menopausal Women" (paper presented at the Annual Scientific Meeting of the Australasian Menopause Society, Auckland, October 1998).

10. M. N. Cayen et al., "Studies on the Disposition of Diosgenin in Rats, Dogs, Monkeys, and Man," *Atherosclerosis* 33 (1979): 71–87.

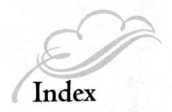

Index